Head Trauma

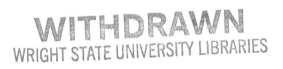

Head Trauma Educational Reintegration

Christine Duncan Rosen, Ph.D.

Principal of the Kennedy Institute
School for Children with Learning Disabilities

Joan P. Gerring, M.D.

Assistant Professor of Child Psychiatry
Johns Hopkins University School of Medicine
Kennedy Institute for Handicapped Children
Baltimore, Maryland

College-Hill Press, San Diego, California

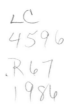
College-Hill Press, Inc.
4284 41st Street
San Diego, California 92105

Library of Congress Cataloging in Publication Data
Main entry under title:

Rosen, Christine Duncan, 1929–
   Head trauma.

   Bibliography: p.
   Includes indexes.
   1. Brain-damaged children—Education—United States.
2. Brain-damaged children—Rehabilitation—United States.
I. Gerring, Joan P., 1943–   . II. Title. [DNLM: 1. Brain
Injuries—in adolescence. 2. Brain Injuries—in infancy &
childhood. 3. Rehabilitation. WS 340 R813h]
LC4596.R67   1986   371.91′6   86-6784

ISBN 0-88744-197-1
Printed in the United States of America

Dedication

To the head trauma children who were patients at the J.F. Kennedy Institute from 1981 to 1984 and their families, from whom I've learned a lot about grief, love, hope, and courage.

Christine Duncan Rosen

To Julia and Judy.

Joan P. Gerring

Acknowledgments

To Jason Brandt, Ph.D. and Lois Pommer, Ed.D., colleagues who reviewed the manuscript.

To Walter Rosen for his support and encouragement.

Christine Duncan Rosen

To Bob Gerring, Jean Christianson, and Lucille McCarthy for support and encouragement and to Yvonne Paige for technical assistance.

Joan P. Gerring

TABLE OF CONTENTS

Introduction

Late one wintry afternoon, a 15 year old boy sped along a bike path toward home. For reasons that can only be suspected, he failed to notice a log across the path and was thrust headlong off the bicycle. The impact of the fall was great enough to cause him to lose consciousness. It is estimated that he lay there more than an hour before being discovered. He experienced 35 days of coma and 3 months of hospitalization before returning home as a partially rehabilitated victim of head injury.

The boy above is one of 20,000 persons under age 21 in this country who have survived a head injury severe enough to have required three weeks or more of hospitalization. He is one of 400,000 persons in the United States who will require long term assistance from society in the form of special education, medical resources, community support in recreation, socialization, job preparation, and probable life-time supervision for many activities. His personality, life style, range of responsibility, career, and social outlook have been drastically altered by a few seconds of inattention or perhaps a misperception of depth. He and many others who have been suddenly and traumatically injured by falls, assaults, and vehicle-involved accidents provide the impetus for writing this book.

Not all head injuries are severe, and not all severe head injuries result in serious losses. But for those whose injuries are both severe and lasting, there are many problems to be addressed. These are problems that involve adequately trained and informed professionals in patients' local communities and the availability of resources that offer psychosocial, medical, educational, and vocational support.

Schools are to children what workplaces are to adults. At the time of hospital discharge, however, children will not have recovered to the extent that one recovers from other illness or disease. In spite of this, families and educational staff can expect many head injured children to return to school, albeit with a modified program.

School work is a central activity for children and the routine, structure, and demand for mental activity made upon students is a critical component of recovery. Support is essential so that there may be success at some level. (No one would expect brain injured adults to return to their former jobs immediately after discharge and carry out tasks as though uninterrupted.) Allowances need to be tempered with expectations and demands in order to maintain a balance between expecting too much and expecting enough.

Head injured children and adolescents will be greatly helped, or hindered, by the responses of adults in the community of schools, churches, temples, Y's, health centers and the workplace. Teachers and others in the educational community, however, fill an especially vital role in restoring the disrupted progress of head injured students to a status more resembling routine and normalcy. School is the most appropriate place for children to gain reassurance that achievement is possible again, even while being confronted with enormous new difficulties in thinking, remembering, speaking, reading, or concentrating.

The chapters that follow will discuss in detail the following conclusions that have been reached by the authors:

- Public Law 94-142 provides for services to children with brain injury but does not address the particular problems of head trauma.

- Head injured students are unique in many ways and are neither easily described nor easily provided for.
- Methods of special education in use for other handicapping conditions are not always applicable to this population.
- Head injured students re-enter school with deficits from the injury compounded by an extended absence from school.
- The effect of head injury upon academic and social reintegration appears greater upon secondary than on elementary students.
- There are very few educational recreational summer programs which are appropriate for recently discharged head trauma students.

These pages address the major problems associated with education of these students. Because children who are survivors of severe closed head injury are a new population, there are not abundant data to verify the range of outcomes. The literature and findings on adult recovery from head injury and those few studies of child injury that exist offer evidence that the effects differ and that what may be true of head injured adults is not necessarily true of head injured children and adolescents.

This new population owes its existence to a combination of developments. Over the last decade, the availability of emergency vehicles and helicopter transport has greatly reduced the time between injury and medical care. Shock trauma units in large, central hospitals now stand by with highly developed technology and well-trained personnel ready to administer critical and intensive emergency care. Advances in the education and sophistication of personnel and the development of complex technologic equipment have kept pace with expanding medical understanding about injury, coma, and the recovery process. For these reasons, the acute care of head injury made great strides during the 1970s and has resulted in greatly increased survival of patients. Many of the patients alive today would not have survived in an earlier period of time. Survival is not without its irony, however; many patients are left with severe deficits. Thus, more survive, but they do so at the cost of great compromise across a spectrum of physical and mental abilities, and emerge from hospitals with severe problems that the community of educators, health workers and families must address.

The discussion and recommendations that follow are based on the authors' observations and experience as members of a pediatric rehabilitation team from September 1981 to September 1984. During this period, the Pediatric Rehabilitation Unit of The Kennedy Institute for Handicapped Children in Baltimore, Maryland, served 165 children and adolescents with head and spinal cord injuries in ages from infancy to 21; 60 with severe closed head injury were eligible to return to school. The total population included patients with other brain disorders such as encephalitis, stroke, open injuries such as gunshot wounds, and spinal cord injuries. All of these are excluded from the conclusions in this book because the effects are quite different from those of closed head injury. Of those patients who returned to school, all required some level of educational intervention and 30 percent were given special services. Although the clinical course and educational experiences of *this* group form the bases for the judgments and conclusions here, it is believed that this group is representative of the general population of children and adolescents who have experienced severe closed head injury. As has been stated, the population of survivors of severe head injury is approximately 10 years old and, therefore, a new one on which much has yet to be written. The authors believe that this 3 year experience has provided considerable familiarity with the problems that head injured children and their families face.

Because brain injury so pervades all else, the educational problems of severe closed head injured students are more likely to be appreciated if they are discussed in the context of the medical course that has preceded school reintegration rather than in a vacuum. For all those who work with these students, it is important to learn about where they have been and what they have been through. The reader will be brought along a medical journey of sorts in preparation for the education and management of those students who do eventually leave hospitals to return to school.

Chapter 1

Anatomy of the Brain

The brain is the central organ of the nervous system. The nervous system is the organ system of thought and activity, both voluntary and involuntary. The brain and connected spinal cord compose the central nervous system. The cranial and spinal nerves, along with their associated nerve cell collections called ganglia, compose the peripheral nervous system. The central and peripheral nervous systems are in constant communication with one another and the activity of one is always influenced by the activity of the other.

Nerve tracts may cross from one side of the central nervous system to the other. Ninety percent of the fibers of the pyramidal tract, a motor tract concerned with distal extremity motion, cross to the opposite side in the lower brainstem (Clark, 1975). In this fashion, an activity on one side of the body may be attributed to neuronal control on the opposite side. When focal injury affects a specific cerebral motor area on the left side, then a motor deficit on the right is affected. If the primary motor area controlling hand movement is damaged by a stroke on the left, then the right hand may be paralyzed. From the highest to the lowest levels of the central nervous system, this crossing of fiber tracts keeps both sides of the nervous system interdependent and in constant communication.

The brain consists of two large cerebral hemispheres, the cerebellum and the brainstem (see Fig. 1–1). The right and left cerebral hemispheres are the largest and uppermost part of the brain and are protectively encased in the skull. The hemispheres control the highest functions of thought, memory, language, sensation, and voluntary movements. Although lower animals have cerebral hemispheres, this part of the brain is most highly developed in humans.

The surface of the hemispheres is divided into a series of folds or gyri by furrows called sulci or fissures. Certain of these fissures divide the brain into portions called lobes. The right and left cerebral hemispheres are incompletely divided by the medial longitudinal fissure. At the bottom of the fissure they are joined together by a broad band of connecting fibers called the corpus callosum.

Each hemisphere is divided into four lobes. The frontal lobe lies in front of the central sulcus of Rolando and above the lateral Sylvian fissure. The lateral fissure and the central sulcus are two prominent, easily identified grooves on the lateral cerebral surface. The frontal lobe occupies about the anterior third of the

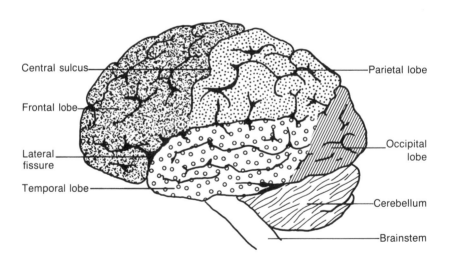

Figure 1–1.   Lateral view of the brain.

hemisphere. Because of its anterior location, it is vulnerable to injury in pedestrian and vehicular trauma. The frontal lobe is the most advanced part of the brain developmentally and contains cells and connections that are not present in lower animals. The frontal lobe contains the primary motor cortex, the supplementary motor areas, and association and projection areas. (Association, projection, and commissural fibers are richly distributed throughout the central nervous system. At every level they connect and interconnect all parts of the system.) The prefrontal cortex is believed to be essential for abstract thinking, language, foresight, mature judgment, and social restraint.

The occipital lobe lies behind a line drawn from the parieto-occipital fissure to the preoccipital notch. The visual cortex and the visual association areas are located here. The parietal lobe extends from the central Rolandic sulcus to the parieto-occipital fissure. Here are located sensory association and projection cortices, as well as speech association areas. Parietal lesions may produce astereognosis, sensory apraxias, and certain kinds of aphasia. (Astereognosis is the inability to recognize an object placed in the hand with the eyes closed. Apraxia is the inability to perform a purposive skilled act, even though the sensory and motor systems are intact.)

The temporal lobe occupies the lateral aspect of the cerebral hemisphere and this location makes it vulnerable to blunt trauma. The portion of the temporal lobe on the lateral surface of the hemisphere lies in front of the occipital lobe, below the lateral fissure and a line extending posteriorly from it to meet the frontal boundary of the occipital lobe (Crosby, Humphrey, and Lauer, 1962). The temporal lobe contains language, auditory, and memory areas. Damage to the temporal lobe may lead to severe memory deficits, hallucinations, and to certain types of seizures.

There are many other important cortical anatomic and functional areas, among which is the limbic lobe, important in the expression of emotions.

The brainstem is connected with the cerebral hemisphere at its rostral end and with the spinal cord at its caudal end. The cerebellum is connected to the brainstem on its dorsal surface. The brainstem consists of all the fiber tracts that exit and enter the cerebral hemispheres. Cell collections within the brainstem are the sensory and motor nuclei of the cranial nerves and other nuclei that regulate voluntary and involuntary activities throughout the body.

The brainstem is divided into the medulla, pons, midbrain and diencephalon. Nuclei in the diencephalon are concerned with the regulation of temperature, heart rate, blood pressure, and appetite. The reticular formation, a collection of cells and fibers extending through the medulla, pons and mesencephalon, is especially important in the regulation of consciousness. The brainstem is a small structure and all of its contents are vital. Any disturbance to the brainstem of either a temporary or permanent nature can cause widespread neurologic impairment because multiple structures are in very close proximity throughout its length. Tumors in the brainstem are often inoperable as even the most delicate surgical effort will lead to damage to important fibers or cells.

The cerebellum is a portion of the brain located under the occipital lobe and attached to the pons, medulla, and midbrain. It is involved with the maintenance of muscle tone and equilibrium and with coordination of movement of muscle groups. Damage to the cerebellum results in ataxia, impaired balance, and decreased muscle tone.

The neuron or nerve cell is the basic unit of the nervous system. It consists of a nerve cell body and cell processes called axons and dendrites. Axons are nerve cell processes that transmit impulses away from the cell body. Dendrites are the nerve processes that transmit impulses toward the cell body. A nerve cell has one axon and one to many dendrites. In the cerebrum and cerebellum, nerve cells are arranged in extensive laminated sheets. Other nerve cell bodies are grouped together in cell collections called nuclei or ganglia. These nerve cell collections are gray in appearance and are referred to as gray matter. Most nerve processes or fibers are encased in a sheath of myelin that is white in color. The remaining brain is therefore termed white matter.

A brain cell in the cerebral gray matter may have processes that extend to a nerve cell in the lower part of the spinal column. The nerve processes of the second neuron travel in a peripheral nerve to a muscle that it innervates. Or the nervous impulse may pass through several neurons as it moves from its origin to the organ that it innervates. Nerve processes also originate in the various organs to transmit messages back to the brain. Nerve circuits are thereby established that provide for a continual interchange of information between the brain and its peripheral connections.

Conduction usually occurs in one direction at the nerve cell synapse. The synapse is the area where the fine processes of one neuron are in contact with the fine processes of another neuron. An impulse travels from dendrite through nerve cell body through axon. At the synapse, a neurotransmitter is released in the form of a vesicle into the synaptic cleft. This vesicle then produces or inhibits an impulse in the dendrites of the adjacent neuron by a process called cell depolarization. In this manner the impulse travels from cell to cell.

Afferent fibers conduct impulses toward the cell body of the neuron; efferent fibers conduct impulses away from the cell body of the neuron. Nerve fibers in the brain and spinal cord that have a common origin and a common destination are called tracts. The cranial and spinal nerves consist of both afferent and efferent fibers. Efferent nerve fibers transmit impulses from the central nervous system to peripheral organs. Efferent fibers terminate in muscles and glands and their discharge results in muscle activation or hormone secretion. Afferent nerve fibers transmit sensory impulses from peripheral organs back to the central nervous system.

When the brain is damaged, deficits stem from injury to those areas of the brain that govern the involved functions. The injury of a missile, as in open head injury, is discrete and brain areas in the path of injury will be affected with predictable deficits. If a bullet passes through the right parietal motor strip, then paralysis of structures on the left side of the body will result.

Blunt injury, on the other hand, results in more diffuse brain damage. Primary damage occurs to structures at the point of impact. Damage may also occur at the point opposite the impact point as the brain is pushed against the interior of the skull. This injury at the point opposite is referred to as the contrecoup injury. Secondary injury results from processes of vasodilation, edema, and increased intracranial pressure that occur as a result of the primary injury. If the right parietal motor strip is at the point of impact, then a left-sided paralysis may occur. A right-sided or bilateral paralysis, however, may result as a consequence of the contrecoup injury or of the more generalized secondary injury.

Chapter **2**

Early Recovery

In casual conversation, the driver of a state of Maryland emergency vehicle explains how medics determine to which hospital accident victims are rushed. "If they look like teenagers, we bring them to the University of Maryland Shock Trauma Unit; if younger, to Johns Hopkins." Both hospitals maintain shock trauma units designed especially for quick response to severe emergencies. Indeed, acute care of closed head trauma is best carried out at large, central referral hospitals because only such hospitals have the equipment, personnel, and facilities to provide the necessary high level of care. The speed with which an individual is transported to an intensive care center is a critical step in modifying the pathological chain of events that stem from the initial injury of impact. Further, the availability of highly skilled emergency personnel and sophisticated medical equipment profoundly alters the course of recovery and effects of injury.

Consider the substance and texture of the brain and its protective structure, the skull. The brain is the consistency of stiff gelatin. The skull, designed to protect the brain from external, penetrating injury, is a bony, hard shell. Inside the skull are uneven protruberances against which the gelatinous mass is forced during a sudden impact. When a car moving at 60 mph stops suddenly against an abutment, another car, or a tree, this soft mass of gelatinous tissue—also traveling at 60 mph until this time—slams against the unforgiving, hard, protrusive interior of a passenger's skull, tearing and shearing the tissue internally.

As Kolb and Whishaw (1980) point out, the brain can be seriously injured from a sudden impact or blows to the head whether or not the skull is fractured, and conversely, skull fracture is not necessarily accompanied by brain damage.

IMMEDIATE EMERGENCY PROCEDURES

Neurologic and respiratory status is assessed quickly when accident victims are brought into an emergency room. Medical personnel first determine whether the person's airway is obstructed and if so, insert a tube into the trachea, or windpipe, to facilitate breathing. (This surgical opening into the trachea is called a tracheostomy.) They also must control bleeding and determine the extent of multiple injuries. Monitoring of all vital signs and pertinent medical functions begins immediately, including systemic and intracranial blood pressure, heart rate, and respiratory rate. Unconscious patients are frequently aided in breathing by respirators that control the quantity of gases that reach the lungs by regulating the depth and duration of breathing. Frequent blood gas analyses measure the amount of oxygen and carbon dioxide in the blood and the pH. All of these parameters are recorded frequently with flow charts that are invaluable in tracking progress or deterioration; the charts also note the effects of multiple medications that are administered. An assessment of overall functioning is given in a Glasgow score.

Glasgow Coma Scale: a measure of the depth and duration of unconsciousness. See page 12 for a longer discussion.

DIAGNOSIS OF INJURY

Significant improvements in medical technology are responsible for improved care and survival of patients. One of the key techniques is called Computerized Tomography or CT scanning.

A CT scan gives important information concerning the presence of edema (swelling) and the presence of any blood clots that may have to be removed surgically. Thus diagnoses of brain pathology can be made within minutes of a patient's entering the hospital. This rapid diagnosis of intracranial bleeding or hematomas (blood collections) is crucial in determining a treatment plan, for there is great danger of excessive blood putting sufficient pressure on brain structures to cause further damage and eventual death.

> The CT scanner was developed by Hounsfield (1973). This advanced X-ray gives a computerized three-dimensional representation of the contents of the skull. It is an extremely valuable diagnostic tool which is noninvasive (i.e., diagnosis is not dependent on an instrument's entering the patient's head). The CT scanner does not identify abnormalities such as epilepsy, but assesses types of brain disruption and atrophy.

Before the development of the CT scanner, clinical judgment played a major role in the decision to perform exploratory surgery to determine the presence of blood clots. In addition, medications known to be effective for control of intracranial pressure were withheld because of their potential to distort the evolving clinical picture. Now, because data obtained from the CT scan are not influenced by different medications, treatment is not affected.

The CT scan also reveals disruption of brain substance, general or localized brain swelling, and areas of bleeding. If a series of CT scans is given, evidence of cerebral changes such as atrophy, enlarged ventricles, and localized brain defects may become more apparent.

IMMEDIATE EFFECTS OF INJURY: INTRACRANIAL PRESSURE

The brain often swells after injury because the disruption causes an increased flow of blood and edema fluid. If the rise in intracranial pressure and edema fluid is not controlled, the patient runs an increased risk of death, for there is no place for release in the confines of the skull. If the swelling is extreme, the brain outgrows the cranial cavity and moves outward and downward in a process called "herniation." This damages the centers of breathing and circulatory regulation in the brainstem and results in death (Fig. 2–1).

> Edema: Excessive accumulation of fluid in cells or in tissue spaces. The fluid comes from the blood capillaries and consists of a clear liquid portion of the blood.

The emergency management of closed head injury consists of treatments to control acute brain swelling and intracranial pressure. A variety of mechanical means and drug treatments are used to decrease cerebral blood flow, reduce and remove edema fluid, and lower intracranial pressure. Common treatments include hyperventilation, corticosteroids, diuretics, barbiturates, and head elevation with head positioned in the midline (Bruce et al., 1979). Raised intracranial pressure (ICP) is much more likely when the initial Glasgow Coma Scale is low (3 or 4). Eighty percent of a series of 35 children with Glasgow scores of 3 or 4 had elevations of intracranial pressure with the pressure rise occurring between the first and fifth postinjury days

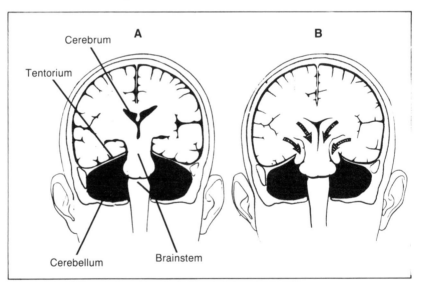

Figure 2–1.   Central transtentorial herniation. *A* shows normal brain relationships in a coronal section. The tentorium is a tough connective tissue membrane separating the cerebral hemispheres from the cerebellum. *B*. As a result of traumatic brain swelling, the cerebral hemispheres expand to compress and displace brainstem structures. This pressure and displacement of vital brainstem areas lead to pathologic circulatory and respiratory changes that may terminate in death. Modified from Plum and Posner, 1980. Reprinted with permission.

(Bruce et al., 1979). While intracranial pressure is elevated, hypothermia, a reduction of body temperature, can be added to the aforementioned treatments. When elevated, the intracranial pressure may remain so for several days. Elevated levels of intracranial pressure and reduction in blood flow result in decreased amounts of oxygen to tissues resulting in focal tissue impairment (Bruce, 1983).

Hypothermia: The purposeful lowering of the body temperature to slow brain metabolism. This depression of brain metabolism may be protective to the brain when oxygen delivery is impaired.

IMMEDIATE EFFECTS OF INJURY: COMA

The monograph *Stupor and Coma*, first published in 1966 by Plum and Posner, focused increased attention on the process of coma or unconsciousness. Before this time, the medical staff gave supportive care to comatose patients and then waited for the clinical course to evolve. Plum and Posner (1966) urged physicians to observe eye signs and breathing patterns of the comatose patient for clues concerning depth and duration of coma. As the sequence of the comatose process became clearer, attention and specific therapy were directed to each step of the process.

Allied Health Professionals: The operation of sophisticated medical equipment has called for new professionals such as respiratory therapists and CT scan/ultrasound technicians. They have become allied with specialty nurses in their goal: to provide optimum treatment as members of an acute care interdisciplinary team. As health care professionals, they are on call day and night to meet patients' needs for critical service and to provide maintenance for their apparatus. Because of the demand for multiple disciplines and because of the extreme attention such patients require, the personnel-to-patient ratio is very high. When a patient with multiple severe injuries is admitted to such a hospital, one nurse is assigned to that patient's care only, and is assisted continually by members of the team.

Patients who suffer severe closed head injury become comatose or unconscious for brief to very long periods of time. A comatose patient does not respond to the stimulus of voice, but lacking other complications, carries on breathing and blood circulation. However, all faculties indicative of a thinking being are suspended, and the patient does not appear to communicate through movement of limbs, periods of calm followed by agitation, or patterns that resemble a sleep/wake cycle. When

Glasgow Coma Scale: In 1974, Teasdale and Jennett utilized the accumulated knowledge about coma to devise a short, easily administered scale to measure the depth and duration of unconsciousness. Intensive care personnel can also use this scale as a rough indicator of a patient's progress in the intensive care setting. It consists of three components: measures of eye opening, motor ability, and verbal ability. The three measures are added and a patient is given a score from 3 to 15. Patients who have initial scores of 8 or less upon admission to the emergency room are usually admitted to an intensive care unit. Patients with scores greater than 8 are admitted to a neurology or neurosurgical unit where care is not as concentrated or as intense. A Glasgow score from 3 to 8 on admission may be taken as an indication of severe head injury. Some experts view the termination of coma as attainment of a Glasgow score of 9. The scale is shown in Appendix A.

the patient moves eyes or limbs in response to a voiced command, it is an indication that the coma has ended. Most commonly, the end of coma is defined as the patient's attainment of the ability to respond to simple commands (Ommaya, 1966). The command may be as simple as a request to raise a designated finger. Eye opening may precede the termination of coma by many days and muteness may continue for a number of days after the simple command response is attained. Coma duration is an important measure of global damage. Duration is stated in numbers of days or hours, according to the method used. Not everyone agrees on how long an individual must be in a coma in order to classify the injury as severe. A coma duration of 6 hours or longer is a frequently used criterion of severe head injury (Jennett and Teasdale, 1981).

Recovery from Coma

Patients emerge from coma gradually. The longer the coma, the more lengthy the process of emergence. Responses to simple commands, at first inconsistent, become more predictable. Gradually, patients obey more complicated commands. The return of speech is the next landmark, but the onset of speaking is delayed if there is oral motor pathology or complication surrounding a tracheostomy.

IMMEDIATE EFFECTS OF INJURY: POSTTRAUMATIC AMNESIA

Another important measurement of the severity of damage is the duration of posttraumatic amnesia (PTA). Three kinds of amnesia, or periods of time for which there is no conscious memory, are associated with head injury. A patient with *retrograde amnesia* has no memory of the time prior to the injury, whether or not it is followed by a period of coma. A patient with no recollection of the time following the injury and coma suffers from *anterograde amnesia*. There is a relationship between the retrograde and anterograde durations, but retrograde amnesia tends to decrease with time and has not been useful as a prognostic indicator. The duration of retrograde amnesia, most often shorter than anterograde amnesia, is usually measured in minutes or hours.

Russell, working with a series of 200 patients with closed head injury, defined *posttraumatic amnesia* as the period after trauma when the patient is not storing continuous memories (Russell, 1932). PTA includes anterograde amnesia and the length of coma, if it has occurred. Patients are not consistently oriented during this period of time, although they may appear oriented at any one testing. Sometimes they appear to be confused. They may carry on simple conversations and give correct answers to questions, or carry on activities without noticeable change in their regular manner of performance. Posttraumatic amnesia cannot be identified simply by random observation.

The Duration of PTA

Medical personnel have long determined the duration of PTA by asking patients (at any time following emergence from amnesia) when they "woke up" or "came to themselves" (Russell, 1932). Years after injury, people retain a reasonable memory of this measure of severity. By contrast, years after injury, it is often difficult to retrieve records that give an accurate measure of the patient's length of coma. PTA is useful as a measure even in very short durations of coma, including momentary lapses of consciousness. Under such circumstances the concept of PTA helps explain why a patient who had a few minutes of unconsciousness and a few days of PTA is unable to work for several months. The duration of PTA has prognostic importance regarding a number of outcomes. In Guthkelch's study (1979) of 398 head injury cases, it was 6 months before the majority of patients with a PTA lasting between 1 and 7 days had returned to work. Also,

Lishman (1968) noted that patients with longer PTAs had a higher incidence of psychiatric deficits. A prospective study of head injured children and adolescents showed a relationship between permanent IQ deficit and PTAs of at least two weeks (Chadwick, 1981). In cases of minor injuries, the duration of PTA is in direct relation to the duration of post-concussion symptoms (Guthkelch, 1979).

Standard measures beyond the patient's report of "waking up" have been developed to measure the termination of PTA. Posttraumatic amnesia ends when the patient is oriented consistently and continuous memory is restored. This time may be determined by repeated testing of orientation and memory over several days. Because islands of memory exist during the time of PTA, a single testing may show the patient to be oriented, but a follow-up test several hours or a day later may confirm a lack of orientation.

Galveston Orientation and Amnesia Test (GOAT): A 10 item bedside test of orientation and continuous memory that is administered serially to document the return of continuous memory (Levin, O'Donnell, and Grossman, 1979). This test has been adapted for use with children and is called the Children's Orientation and Amnesia Test (COAT). See Appendix B (Ewing-Cobbs et al., 1984). When patients have achieved a certain score on sequential COAT or GOAT testing, they are no longer considered to be in PTA.

Case History

R.S. is a $16\frac{8}{12}$ year old 12th grade female student who suffered severe closed head injury as a driver in an auto accident. Her initial Glasgow score was 8/15 and her CT scan was within normal limits. She was hospitalized in a neurointensive care unit and was comatose for 9 days. The patient was admitted to the rehabilitation hospital on the 22nd day after her injury. The termination of PTA was documented by sequential GOATs and occurred 36 days after injury. During the PTA, R.S. answered "I don't know" to the question "What is the first event you can remember after the injury?" After the PTA ended, she answered, "Waking up at JFK. . . . I thought it was all a dream." Deficits in short term memory persisted after the termination of the PTA.

IMMEDIATE EFFECTS OF INJURY: SEIZURES

Seizures are a common complication of severe head injury. Head trauma patients may experience seizures as a result of their injury. This type of seizure disorder is called posttraumatic epilepsy (PTE). Severe enough injury to the brain causes a disturbance in the electrical rhythms that, in turn, provokes an abnormal electrical discharge. The chances that these seizures will occur with any brain injury are 5 percent. As the severity of injury increases, however, the incidence of seizures rises. Brink, Imbus, and Woo-Sam (1980) describe a group of patients with a medium duration of coma of 5 to 6 weeks, among whom the incidence of seizures was 32 percent.

Epilepsy: A disorder of the nervous system characterized by abnormal discharge of the nerve cells, called a seizure or fit. Seizures may take a variety of forms, from motor movements to abnormal sensory experiences to behaviors such as aggression. Temporary loss of consciousness follows some seizures.

Electroencephalograph (EEG): A measure of electrical activity of the brain, picked up by a standard placement of electrodes on the scalp. Deviation from the usual recorded rhythms over certain brain areas is defined as pathological. Abnormalities include excessively slow or fast activity and certain spike and wave patterns. The EEG may be unremarkable, however, in the presence of brain damage, or may show abnormalities when the patient has no signs or symptoms of illness.

Seizure disorders may take a variety of forms. Seizures may be convulsive, involving motor movements, or non-convulsive in nature. Non-convulsive seizures are the more common disorders and include simple partial and complex partial varieties. When seizures consist completely of mental symptoms, such as fear or depression, they are often difficult to recognize. Simple partial seizures are not usually accompanied by a loss of consciousness. These seizures involve a discharge in one or another area (e.g., movement of an extremity, an abnormal sensation of smell or taste, a hallucination, or the experience of anger). Complex partial seizures may sometimes begin with simple partial symptoms, but are usually accompanied by impaired consciousness (e.g., mild confusion, a haze that comes and goes, or a tendency to stare). Complex partial seizures last about 30 seconds to 3 minutes (Murray, 1985).

Immediately after trauma, the EEG often demonstrates a variety of abnormalities including diffuse or focal slow rhythms. As the distance from trauma lengthens over weeks or months, the EEG often appears more normal. Many patients will eventually have a pattern that is interpreted as normal even though posttraumatic epilepsy may appear later.

Posttraumatic seizures may occur early in the first week following trauma or appear much later. The more severe the trauma, the greater the likelihood of early seizures. When early posttraumatic seizures are present, children are at risk for eventual development of late posttraumatic seizures as well. A more severe injury also increases risk for late seizures that may make their appearance years afterward. Less obvious seizures can seem to be a deterioration in the recovery process. A previously attentive child, for example, may appear disinterested or inattentive if there are numerous seizure discharges unaccompanied by abnormal movements. Although seizures will cease in one half of the patients who develop posttraumatic epilepsy, one quarter to one third of patients will continue to have 10 to 15 seizures a year (Rosman and Oppenheimer, 1982). These seizures are often very difficult to treat.

Some research suggests a prophylactic value for antiseizure medication as part of the early management regimen (Wohns and Wyler, 1979; Young, Rapp, Brooks, Madauss, and Norton, 1979). In institutions subscribing to this preventive measure, all patients with severe injury are treated for a predetermined length of time with anticonvulsants. This treatment is prolonged if seizures develop; then patients are put on a regular maintenance schedule. Conclusive studies regarding the value of this prophylyactic treatment are lacking, however.

The standard treatment of seizures is with medication, but helping a child attain good seizure control requires finding a delicate balance among dosage, blood level toxicity and minimal side effects. All children and adolescents who have had seizures must be followed on a regular basis by a physician. The physician is helped in this endeavor by drug assays performed on blood samples that specify a therapeutic range of drug values. Toxic effects may appear when the medication surpasses the therapeutic range, or even while it still is in the therapeutic range. Common side effects of special concern to the child and adolescent population are sedation and hyperactivity. These behavioral effects may seriously impede classroom performance; indeed, it is often teachers who notice these symptoms. In addition, teachers are in a position to monitor the occurrence of seizures and the behavioral effects of any changes in medication.

IMMEDIATE EFFECTS OF INJURY: OTHER IMPAIRMENT

Physical Problems

Motor Impairment

Diffuse cerebral and brainstem injury results in damage to pathways that regulate movement, posture, and coordination. Spasticity, or exaggerated reflexes to the point of paralysis, may occur on either or both sides of the body. Although the paretic (weakened) side is usually the side opposite the injury, it is not always so. Closed head injury frequently has diffuse effects in other brain areas than the point of impact. These do not always show up on the CT scan.

> Hemiparesis: Weakness on one side of the body (e.g., the right arm and right leg). Muscle reflexes are exaggerated or abnormal on the side of the hemiparesis. Weakness so severe that the patient is unable to move is called paralysis. Paralysis on one side of the body is called hemiplegia.

Patients undergo physical therapy measures early in the intensive care course to prevent muscle contracture or tightening in both upper and lower extremities. When patients are unable to move by themselves, they are positioned and provided with passive exercises to the limbs in order to prevent atrophic changes. Other effects of motor impairment are discussed in detail in Chapter 3. Until a patient emerges from coma, passive therapy and positioning are standard treatment.

Internal Injuries

Internal injuries have long lasting effects and may involve any organ. Rupture of the spleen requires its removal, which in turn makes patients especially vulnerable to infection. Other organs or parts of organs, such as the lungs, liver, kidneys, or bowels, can be so damaged their present or future function is compromised. A lung or bowel segment or an entire kidney may have to be removed if it is damaged, if the blood supply is threatened, or if bleeding is excessive.

Hypertension

Hypertension is another possible complication of severe closed head injury that may persist for weeks or months. The heightened pressure must be controlled by medication. Brink and colleagues (1980) noted 20 percent of 344 patients had hypertension during their rehabilitation hospital course. The most severely impaired patients had the highest incidence of hypertension (46 percent).

Sleeping and Waking Patterns

Sleep/wake cycles are disrupted by injury and medication. During early recovery, the patient may sleep on and off throughout the day and night, not observing the usual day/night sequence. Resumption of the normal sleep/wake cycle is an important indication of improvement.

A patient's activity level is an important biologic indicator, and may be abnormal in a variety of ways. Quiet periods may alternate with periods of random, diffuse, high activity. These high activity periods are of special concern because the patients are a potential danger to themselves and to others. No matter what the level, the activity appears random with a confused, disoriented quality. The activity may be in response to external stimulation; therefore, the more a patient is stimulated by voice or sight or external activity, the greater may be the response of heightened activity. In some patients, the activity level increases to an agitated or aggressive quality.

Agitation

Agitation is defined as extreme restlessness that includes screaming, pacing, and undirected movement of the trunk and limbs. Patients confined to bed may throw themselves restlessly around the bed. They may further injure themselves by hitting hard parts of the bed or by falling on the floor. For this reason, the bed may be padded or a patient's limbs briefly restrained during the height of the agitation. At times the agitation takes on a component of aggression, usually random with an impulsive quality. A patient may strike a caretaker with considerable force or may suddenly throw a glass at a fellow patient. Such patients need special staff attention to insure the safety and protection of themselves and others. Medications are often used during this time.

Occasionally rehabilitation hospital staff is unable to work with a patient who is aggressive. In such a situation, patients are transferred to a psychiatric hospital. In a follow-up study of 70 adult patients, Levin and Grossman (1978) stated that patients who showed agitation in the early stages of recovery from coma were at increased risk for the development of later emotional and behavioral sequelea. In the Kennedy Institute population, patients who went through a stage of prominent agitation often had a premorbid history of behavioral disorder. The posttraumatic behavior at times appears to be an exacerbation of the premorbid behavioral symptom.

Case History

T.H. is an $18\frac{3}{12}$ year old white male who suffered closed head injury with a brainstem and a right hemispheric contusion as a passenger in March 1982. The patient had been hospitalized for a head injury and a brief period of unconsciousness at age 6. Migraine headaches were diagnosed at age 9. T.H. was a poor student with problems starting in the third grade, including aggression and disruptive behavior. Truancy, drinking, and drug abuse became problems in high school. The patient quit high school on his 18th birthday. The patient had been placed on probation three times connected with the destruction of property. T.H. was unconscious for 5 days. Four days after coma ended, aggressive behavior began. He developed a posttraumatic seizure disorder in the 2nd week after injury and was admitted to a rehabilitation hospital 2 months after injury. The patient was verbally and physically aggressive towards staff members. He forcefully threw a glass pestle at the wall, threw a chair at the wall, and hit his nurse in the abdomen. He made several attempts to escape from the hospital. In one attempt, the patient put his leg over a rail on a second floor porch. Thioridazine was used to achieve mild sedation, with a mild decrease in the level of aggression. Because T.H. was a behavioral/psychiatric patient, with limited need for other disciplines, transfer to a psychiatric facility was arranged.

As the patient's vital functions stabilize, from intracranial pressure to heart rate, the need to continuously monitor these functions decreases. Physical and occupational therapists anticipate rehabilitation needs by making visits to the intensive care unit to position patients and to work with muscles that have begun to contract.

There are many severe medical problems that will detain a patient in intensive care. Extracranial injuries accompany head injuries in patients admitted to the hospital in one third of the cases (Jennett and Teasdale, 1981). These problems include severe injury to internal organs necessitating surgery, fractures, massive infections, hypertension, and derangements of the hormonal system. Any one of these problems may contribute to a deterioration or a plateau in the patient's clinical condition. When it is determined that all systems of the patient are no longer in need of constant medical attention, patients are transferred to a neurological or neurosurgical unit for further care.

Psychosocial Problems

The sudden onset of such a severe illness is a great crisis to each family. The possibility of death may exist for several days and the family lives with this uncertainty. At the moment when the dreadful news is delivered, the family struggles to maintain its integrity and well-being, despite grief and fear and anger that are sometimes overwhelming. For several weeks, family life is centered on the crisis. Job schedules are disrupted. Sleep is caught at irregular times. Parents may be troubled by anxiety dreams. Eating is sporadic and the quality of nutrition often falls for family members. Most families have had no preparation for the medical system of advanced technology that they now enter with their child. In a few days' time they are asked to assimilate such terms as CT scan, tracheostomy, and respirator so they may begin to ask important questions concerning management.

Siblings are often in the care of nearby relatives. Depending on their age and the dynamics of the family, they may or may not actively participate in events. However, the lives of most siblings living with the patient are affected by the events of the accident and its aftermath. Because of the magnitude and complexity of tasks addressed by the parents, the questions and needs of siblings are often ignored for a time.

Families show different styles of adaptation to crisis. There is little research concerning an optimal family background for coping with crisis, but several contributors to adaptation have emerged from observation and work with the families of patients at the Kennedy Institute:

- *Stable family background.* A follow-up study by Gilchrist and Wilkinson (1979) found a stable family to be a positive influence on prognosis of 84 adults.
- *Family style.* Family style depends greatly on its interaction with the outside world and may be exaggerated during a crisis. Some families work well with outside helpers and establish a mutual give-and-take relationship. Others are untrusting and isolated and find it difficult to surrender the care of their children to others.
- There are very dependent families that rely heavily on staff guidance and are unable to initiate needed services. The long term outcome of a patient's recovery from an injury does not appear to depend on whether families accept and subscribe to a medical regimen or whether they deny many of the potential problems.
- *Family support.* Psychologic resources are necessary to embark on this long and trying period. Families who lack resources or who have been unable to resolve lesser crises in the past are placed under severe strain and risk deterioration. Social work support is an important adjunct during the inpatient and outpatient periods of recovery.

Families with a strong religious belief find powerful and long-sustaining support during this crisis. In the long run, those families who persevere, continue to hope and are part of a cohesive support system maintain themselves through the difficult rehabilitation period.

Emotional Responses

Anger and *denial* are two common early emotional responses to the injury. Anger, open or suppressed, arises from the incomprehensible nature of the occurrence and the resulting distress of the entire family. Obtaining a lawyer to investigate the circumstances of the accident and initiating litigation are socially acceptable mechanisms for the discharge of angry feelings. Another focus of anger is on medical treatments or personnel. Some parents develop conflicts with particular staff members over various treatment methods. Other parents will focus on an aspect of the hospital environment that they find troublesome. One mother became concerned that her child would further injure herself while agitated by hitting herself against the sides of her metal bed. The mother spent several weeks making padded cloth bedliners until she felt satisfied that one was effective. Staff members must analyze each expression of parental dissatisfaction to separate the real and present issues from the diffuse and projected responses stemming from feelings about the accident.

Families frequently deny the severity of the injury as explained by medical or rehabilitation staff. For example, families of patients who have experienced many weeks of coma and who continue to show severe resultant handicaps will talk about college attendance as an imminent occurrence. Attempts to dissuade such families are futile. Sometimes family denial seriously interferes with rehabilitation. Parents may relate to the child as if there were no handicap and make no attempt to contribute to or support the treatment effort. Such parents delay certain schedules by not implementing treatment plans during home visits.

Such denial frequently lessens as the time from injury lengthens. Although parents may continue to maintain that their child will recover without handicap, most increasingly subscribe to treatment recommendations. In such instances, denial may be viewed as initial protection against the severe psychologic stress. With time most families gain some mastery of their new situation and no longer have to use denial to keep severe tension under control.

Other emotions are prominent in different individuals. Depression and anxiety may appear in family members who have a predisposition toward those conditions. Most often the appearance and resolution of strong feelings are managed within the family with assistance and support of friends, neighbors, and church. When the emotional reaction of parents negatively affects a patient's treatment or if parents are unable to reduce levels of tension with the assistance of their own social network, then intervention is offered. Hospital personnel, mindful that personality traits tend to be temporarily exaggerated during crises, do not suggest counseling or therapy until a reasonable estimate can be made of the persistence of maladaptive patterns of behavior. When families are isolated, or when there is severe family dysfunction, early intervention in the form of crisis management is usually attempted by the social work or psychiatric staff.

SUMMARY

The period of time from injury to the end of the posttraumatic amnesia is packed with events and emotional reaction to these events. This period is measured in weeks and months. Advanced technology insures the survival of most patients who arrive at the intensive care unit. As the comatose condition subsides, rehabilitation efforts are directed toward the deficits that become apparent. Each rehabilitation specialist periodically assesses the pattern of recovery and the prominent deficits in his area of interest. As soon as the patient has the mental capacity to incorporate new material, these specialists institute treatment strategies. At the termination of posttraumatic amnesia, patients have received a complete assessment of deficits and have embarked on comprehensive programs for their alleviation. For those patients who do not receive inhospital rehabilitation, the termination of the PTA may mark the time to re-enter the community.

Chapter **3**

Long Term Recovery

It is common for patients to be still comatose and in posttraumatic amnesia when they leave intensive care units. At that time, patients are no longer on respirators and can breathe on their own (although with tracheostomies, for some) and they no longer hover between life and death. Much medical and nursing care is still needed, but that care can be given at a less costly and less extensively monitored setting than an intensive care unit.

At the end of posttraumatic amnesia (PTA), which may be days to months after injury, patients are consistently oriented to place, date, and time and are able to store long term memories. It is then that the most productive rehabilitation begins. The rate of recovery in physical and cognitive areas is greatest in the year following injury. For this reason, many patients will spend several weeks or months in a progression of hospital settings, from intensive care to a general neurological or surgical ward, and then to a rehabilitation hospital. When patients are ready to leave the general hospital, they are often unable to go directly home. Many are still dependent for most aspects of their care. They may not yet be able to walk, feed, or clean themselves or control bladder or bowels. Still other patients continue with serious medical complications such as tracheostomy dependency or complicated, slowly healing fractures. Early behaviors such as agitation and aggression often make discharge to home during early recovery impractical if not impossible.

> Rehabilitation: Graduated programs of physical and mental exercises to encourage return of damaged functions. These programs are devised and administered by trained professionals in physical, cognitive, and psychologic specialities.

The role of rehabilitation in the early recovery period is unclear. Physical therapy is known to have a beneficial role in the prevention and alleviation of contractures; but whether rehabilitation influences the return of motor abilities, cognition, or speech prior to termination of PTA is not known.

Rehabilitation efforts have a more apparent role when patients demonstrate the capacity to store and retrieve new information. During the early stages of PTA, patients are provided with family photos and familiar belongings such as stuffed animals or blankets. They are encouraged to participate in a daily group activity of identifying who they are, where they are, and what has happened to develop orientation to the setting. Orientation to the date and time follows and continues throughout the period of PTA.

While no one asserts that rehabilitation efforts have certain effects, that ongoing recovery from head injury does occur is well documented. According to Chadwick, Rutter, Brown, Shaffer, and Traub (1981), cognitive gains continue in the second year after trauma, but at a reduced rate. Lewin, Marshall, and Roberts (1979) state that recovery of children and adolescents after severe head injury continues for five years. It is logical to assume, with further technologic advances in neurointensive care and increased survival, that the quality of survival will improve and the duration of healing lengthen. Despite average durations, rehabilitation clinicians are accustomed to exceptional cases of restoration or great improvement in a specific function months or years after healing has leveled off.

Case History

D.P. is an 18 year old white male who suffered severe closed head injury with a right parietal depressed skull fracture and a right parietal hematoma in an assault at age $15\frac{1}{2}$. The patient was comatose for 5 weeks. Tracheostomy and gastrostomy were necessary during his intensive care course. Eighteen months after injury, the patient had a left hemiparesis, dysarthria, and impaired swallowing. Muscle tone was significantly increased in the left leg with an equinovarous deformity and a 20 degree heel cord contracture. D.P. needed a cane and a left short leg brace to assist walking. A Tendo-Achilles Lengthening Procedure was performed 2 years after injury to relieve the heel cord contracture and to improve ambulation. Two and one-half years after injury no neurologic or functional improvement had been noted. Physical therapy services were discontinued. The next Kennedy follow-up occurred 3½ years after injury. Tone in the left lower extremity had decreased to where the patient was able to utilize the muscle strength in his ankle for greatly improved ambulation. Cane and brace were no longer necessary.

Klonoff, Low, and Clark (1977) obtained initial and annual EEGs as one aspect of their prospective 5 year follow-up of head injured children. Other aspects that were examined were neuropsychologic function, neurologic status and school progress. One hundred thirty-one patients were younger than 9 years at the time of injury and 100 patients were older than 9 years. The EEGs of the older children had stabilized by 3 years after trauma, while improvement was still evident in the younger group 5 years after trauma. On the fifth re-examination there was still evidence of EEG abnormality in 15 percent of the younger group and 5 percent of the older group. No specific EEG abnormality showed any particular correlation with seizures. Of the sample of both younger and older children, 76.3 percent made a marked recovery over time. Recovery extended over the whole 5 years because significant contrasts were still found between the fourth and fifth follow-up examinations. The most important prognostic variables were the initial full scale IQ and the duration of coma.

The relationship of coma to long term effects has been demonstrated in two controlled prospective studies of cognitive recovery in children and adolescents after severe closed head injury. The study by Chadwick and coworkers (1981) extended for 2¼ years and tracked children who were between ages 5 and 14 at the time of injury. The severe head injury group consisted of 31 children with PTA of at least 1 week, while the mild head injury group consisted of 29 children with a history of PTA of 1 hour to less than 1 week. The control group included 28 children hospitalized with accidental orthopedic injuries. No evidence of persistent cognitive damage was found when PTA was less than 24 hours, but with PTAs of 3 or more weeks, there were persistent intellectual deficits at the 2¼ year follow-up. The authors concluded that intellectual impairment showed a positive relationship to the duration of PTA.

No prospective studies of cognitive and neuropsychologic recovery extend beyond 5 years. There are two follow-up studies of small numbers of young patients who suffered long periods of coma after severe head injury. Richardson (1963) reported on 10 patients ages 5 to 18 at the time of their injuries. Median duration of coma was 28 days, with a range from 7 to 47 days. Median duration of PTA was 49 days, with a range from 25 to 65 days. Follow-up duration ranged from 2 to 14 years, with all patients followed for at least 2 years. Patients showed a loss of from 10 to 30 IQ points from their estimated level of intelligence at preinjury. Each patient showed a larger range of variation in individual tests and subtests than is usually found in a normal population. All the patients performed poorly on tests of rote memory. Perseveration, poor comprehension, and concreteness were specifically noted as intellectual deficits.

Another long term retrospective follow-up series of severely injured children and adolescents was published by Brink, Garrett, Hale, Woo–Sam, and Nickel (1970). Forty-six patients from the Rancho Los Amigos Hospital were evaluated 1 to 7 years after severe head injury. These patients were ages 2 to 18 at the time of their admission to this rehabilitation hospital. Three patients had been comatose for longer than 1 year, but the average duration of coma for patients who regained consciousness was 7 weeks, with a median duration of 4 weeks. All of the patients showed a decrease in IQ from preinjury status in follow-up examinations. Thirty-three percent of the 46 patients scored within the normal level, 30 percent were borderline retarded, 23 percent were mildly retarded, 9 percent were moderately retarded, and 5 percent were severely retarded. Brink and coworkers documented a direct relationship between the length of coma and the follow-up IQ. Their findings agree with Chadwick's. Patients who tested in the normal range of intelligence had an average coma duration of 1.7 weeks; those who tested in the borderline range had an average coma duration of 3 weeks.

Patients who tested in the mildly retarded range had an average coma duration of 8 weeks, while patients who tested in the severely retarded range had an average coma duration of 11 weeks.

NEED FOR CONTINUING REHABILITATION

Thus far studies have shown that recovery continues for many years and that the longer the coma, the greater the damage. It is believed by rehabilitative, multidisciplinary staff that therapies are critical during the period of rapid change, usually within the 1st year after injury. In fact, the amount of therapy is often determined by how rapidly the patient is changing and usually decreases as the rate of change decreases. In a British survey by Gilchrist and Wilkinson (1979), those adult patients in a coma from 24 hours to 1 week required 6 months of rehabilitation. Those unconscious 2 to 7 weeks required nearly a year of rehabilitation, and those unconscious 8 weeks or more required nearly 2 years of rehabilitation. All of this rehabilitation does not have to go on in a hospital, and in fact the rising costs of medical care curtail lengthy stays and make it necessary for consumers to turn to outpatient care. Medically stable patients with decreasing needs for therapy are discharged to home, where needed services are found in the community. (More will be said about transitions to home and school in Chapter 4.) Rehabilitation does continue for a long time, and much of it is carried out in a hospital setting. The average length of stay for the Kennedy Institute population was 2 months.

As the patient's medical condition stabilizes, patient management is assumed by a multidisciplinary rehabilitation team, usually with a physiatrist in charge. Their efforts concentrate on the medical/physical aspects of recovery, as these aspects improve most rapidly and their treatment fits well into a medical hospital setting. Many disciplines make up the rehabilitative team: medicine and nursing, neurology and neuropsychology, psychiatry, orthopedic surgery and dentistry, occupational and physical therapy, speech-language pathology, audiology, recreational therapy, social work, education, nutrition, and clinical and behavioral psychology. At first medical care is intensive, but as the patient's condition improves, the emphasis shifts from physical rehabilitation to cognitive, behavioral, and psychosocial rehabilitation.

CONTINUING MEDICAL PROBLEMS

The performance of a tracheostomy during the acute course is an indication of the severity of the injury. This procedure is not done unless a patient is unable to breath independently or to attain a sufficient quantity of oxygen in the lungs for a prolonged period of time. Fifty-five percent of the patients in the series by Brink and colleagues (1980) received an early tracheostomy. A decision to perform a tracheostomy is a most serious one, for tracheostomy care is delicate and difficult. Fastidious care, including the use of monitoring equipment, must be taken to insure that the patient's airway remains open and that the delivery of gases is unimpeded. When the patient's clinical condition improves, attempts are made to close the tracheostomy opening gradually so that the patient can resume breathing in the regular manner. Plugs and progressively smaller tubes are used so that the opening becomes smaller and eventually closes, leaving a scar. Occasionally a patient unable to tolerate the withdrawal of oxygen or the closing of the tracheostomy will continue to be tracheostomy dependent for an indeterminate length of time. Facial and skin scarring or disfigurement are medical complications with great psychologic import. Multiple facial scars or a tracheostomy scar with heavy discolored scar tissue can be very unsightly.

Facial fractures are the most common extracranial injury. These fractures may heal in an asymmetric manner and cause disfigurement. In all such instances, the plastic surgeon and the oral surgeon are consulted early in the clinical course to submit a sequential plan for scar removal and degrees of facial reconstruction. A face paralyzed on one side, a drooping eyelid, or missing teeth draw negative attention to a patient.

Ataxia: Disturbance of the coordination of the muscular movements.

Damage to the cerebellum and to the sensory tracts that regulate coordination of movement will result in impaired balance, tremors, and dysarthric speech. A patient's balance often improves early in recovery, but an ataxic gait sometimes persists. This gait has a staggering quality and is occasionally misinterpreted as drunkenness; a former patient from the Kennedy Institute was arrested after a minor motor vehicle accident because police believed he was intoxicated. Tremors also frequently improve, persisting only to a minor degree. Occasionally an intention tremor of the upper limbs will be handicapping enough to prevent functional use of the hand for fine movements. The patient, for example, may be unable to hold a full cup of liquid without spilling it.

Ataxic speech is termed "dysarthric," and has a scanning, slurred quality. Ataxia was seen in 60 percent of the 52 patients followed by Brink and colleagues (1980), but the majority of these patients were affected to a minimum degree.

Physical ailments may slow the recovery process. Orthopedic injuries, mainly extremity fractures, complicate the problems of spasticity and ataxia, thereby slowing attainment of arm or leg function. A fracture of the humerus prevents an aggressive program of therapy on a contracted, paralyzed arm. A fracture of the femur may require traction for several weeks, prolonging the time until the patient can progressively attain ambulation. A leg fracture complicated by numerous breaks or impaired healing may result in uneven leg length and a limp. Relearning to write or walk requires not only neurologic healing in the areas of the brain that control motor function but also orthopedic healing of bones and tissue.

Spasticity

In many patients spasticity is at first severe and then decreases. When leg spasticity is severe, patients are unable to walk. As spasticity lessens, progressive physical therapy exercises are instituted to prepare patients for the resumption of walking.

When arm spasticity is severe, patients are unable to use the arm and hand. Along with passive exercises, the occupational therapist may use splinting to prevent muscle tightening. As arm spasticity lessens, progressive exercises to restore strength to muscles of the arm and hand are instituted. Moderate spasticity may result in awkward fine motor movements. When spasticity is severe and the arm is paralyzed with contracted muscles, then the arm and hand may remain motionless at the side with the arm flexed at the elbow. If the right hand and arm are irreversibly affected in a right-handed individual, the occupational therapist begins work with the patient to change handedness.

Although hyperactive reflexes persisted in 93 percent of patients in a follow-up study by Brink and colleagues (1970), functional use of both arms and legs was restored in most patients. In this series, only three patients who regained consciousness remained unable to walk after an average follow-up of 1 to 7 years.

Bracing and canes may be used in preparation for independent walking. When the patient begins to walk again, a limp may still remain, or exaggerated reflexes may be the only residual damage.

COGNITIVE AND LANGUAGE PROBLEMS

Mental impairment is the most troublesome effect of head injury. From the time of the injury, severe diffuse derangement results in global impairment of all areas of functioning. The most extreme aspect of this derangement is the comatose state described earlier. When patients first emerge from coma, there is little evidence that cognitive faculties are working. A patient may be responsive to voice and may obey simple commands. Attempts to elicit more evidence of cognitive functioning may be too stimulating to the damaged nervous system and a patient may respond with increased motor activity. Gradually, depending on the severity of the injury and the subsequent clinical course, cognitive abilities return over days to months. Each day may signal the return of a new function. The return of speech follows emergence from coma by a few days. At first the patient will say a word or two; then simple phrases and sentences follow in hours or days. The patient C.M. illustrates this process.

Case History

C.M. was a $10\frac{9}{12}$ year old black male, a fifth grade student at the time of his head injury as a pedestrian. The patient remained comatose for 36 days. Forty-six days after injury, the patient began saying words like "Yes" and "No" and phrases like "Hi, Mom."

By the next day the patient was saying more words and repeating names of people. By 50 days after injury, sentence length had increased to several words (e.g., "I have to go to school."). The patient was able to obey more complex one and two step commands, but continued to be disoriented to time and place. The posttraumatic amnesia ended 65 days after injury. By this date, C.M. was demonstrating increased initiation of spoken communication.

Restoration of cognitive functions seems to follow a progression similar to the initial speech and language development of a young child (i.e., from simple receptive understanding to word usage to increasingly complex phrases). Sometimes oral-motor dysfunction impedes the resumption of speech. This dysfunction may be secondary to cranial nerve damage or to local pathology such as the build-up of fibrous tissue around a tracheostomy scar. Such dysfunction, termed "communicative dissonance," may be temporary and is estimated to occur in about 10 percent of the severe closed head injury population. Assistance is given to these patients as soon as it is determined that their level of general intelligence is high enough to profit from a communication device. D.K. is a patient who received treatment for his severe speech dysfunction.

Case History

D.K. is a 25 year old white male who suffered severe closed head injury as a passenger in an automobile. He remained comatose for 10 weeks. Deficits 1 year after injury included severe right hemiplegia, moderate left hemiparesis, and paralysis of cranial nerves 9, 10, 11, and 12. D.K. was unable to speak and swallow, and his head control was poor. Receptive vocabulary, word retrieval, and recent memory were impaired. Full scale WAIS IQ was 75.

Fifteen months after injury, D.K. was transferred to the Kennedy Institute (Fig. 3–1). With residual left hand function, he had already learned how to use a Canon Communicator (Fig. 3–2). His printed output was characterized by multiple spelling errors and disorganized sentences. He was also proficient in the use of an alphabet board.

The primary goal of the adminission was to develop use of a communication system which would be most appropriate to D.K.'s abilities and needs. A related goal was to improve the

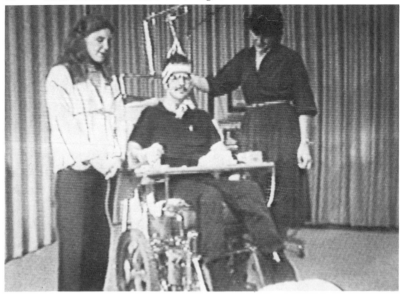

Figure 3–1. D.K. in motorized wheelchair with head support apparatus. Wheelchair controls and Canon Communcator sit on wheelchair tray.

quality of the patient's interactional skills within a variety of settings. D.K. was seen for 7 to 10 hourly individual sessions weekly, in addition to daily group sessions. His parents also participated in his program. During his 6 month admission, he was trained in the use of various supplemental and alternative means of communication. These systems included a Sharp memowriter, a handheld communication device with a typed print-out and a 40-item memory storage unit. D.K. was trained in communicative use of an Apple computer (Fig. 3–3). Supplemental hardware provided either printed or vocal output of messages typed into the computer. D.K. also learned to use the Vocaid, a portable device with voice output. The patient was also trained in the production of signs and gestures with his left hand. At the time of his discharge the memowriter was the preferred device. This device was attached to his wheelchair tray or to a tray across his bed. He became proficient in typing with the device and in programming and accessing its memory.

Communication Devices: Such instruments range in sophistication. The choice of instrument is determined by the physical and mental ability of the patient, the cost of the device, and the predicted duration of the deficit. An alphabet board with a pointer may be used on a short term basis. Sometimes a typewriter is placed on a tray over the patient's wheelchair or patients are equipped with computer keyboards. Some of these computer systems are equipped with a voice to facilitate communication by making it a more rapid and more natural process.

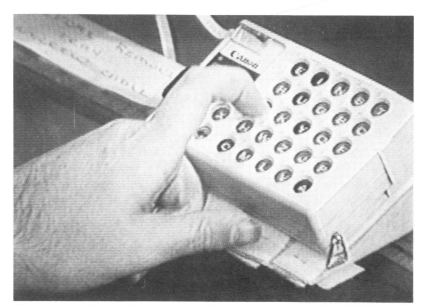

Figure 3–2. Canon Communicator in use.

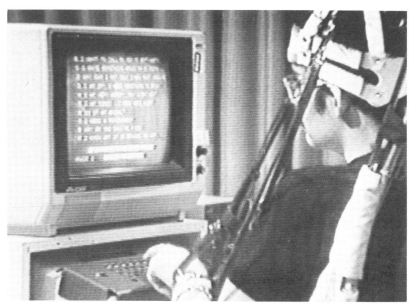

Figure 3–3. D.K. uses the Apple computer as a communication device.

Once a patient can communicate, cognitive, motor and psychologic recovery can be more easily defined. A particular pattern of deficits becomes more apparent. For example, patients may act disoriented in regard to location and to time, but the extent of disorientation can only be estimated until logical spoken sentences are used and lack of orientation is conveyed. At this time they often reveal emotional reactions of fear or anxiety or lack of information about where they are or what has happened to them.

Language dysfunction following injury is a result of global cognitive damage, wherein language is viewed as a function of cognition and is therefore determined by it. However, language deficits may also result from focal damage to the areas of the brain that govern speech and oral-motor activity (dysarthria) or language areas (aphasia). Whether treating language dysfunction as primary language pathology or as secondary to a more global deficit, therapists track individual recovery and use treatments that foster expressive and receptive use of language.

Dysarthria is a defect in the oral-motor aspects of speech, which include articulation, stress, resonance, and intonation. *Aphasia* is a group of deficits in the use of speech for purposes of expression and reception of language. Aphasia is defined and classified by administration of a battery of tests such as the Multilingual Aphasia Examination or the Neurosensory Center Comprehensive Examination for Aphasia. If a person lacks an overt language deficit, yet performs poorly on any of the subtests of an aphasia battery, then subclinical aphasia is presumed. Sarno (1980) studied 56 adult patients 3 months after severe closed head injury (CHI) using 4 of the 20 subtests from the Neurosensory CEB Battery: Visual Naming, Word Fluency, Sentence Repetition, and the Token Test. The entire study population showed a significant degree of verbal impairment in that 32 percent were aphasic, 38 percent were dysarthric with subclinical aphasia, and 30 percent of the group were subclinically aphasic. Subtest scores of the subclinical group ranged from the 72nd to the 79th percentile on the aphasia profile. These outcomes are indicative of serious deficits in either expressive or receptive language abilities.

Aphasia is difficult to characterize and follow in childhood, as the process of development influences the definition of linguistic problems as well as the recovery process.

Muteness is often present in patients for several days after emergence from coma, but with resumption of speech, the most common linguistic disturbance is *anomia*, a defective naming of objects. In addition, slow speech, reduced associative fluency, and circumlocution are present. In comparable populations, Levin and Eisenberg (1979) found linguistic deficits in one third of children and adolescents, but in one half of the adults studied. Only one third of his study population had been comatose for more than 24 hours. Although early neuropsychologic impairment was found in patients with coma of less than 24 hours, persistence of intellectual deficit to about the end of the first year after injury was confined to patients who were comatose longer than 24 hours.

Some speech and language pathologists such as Hagen (1981) believe that the prominent language disorganization following head trauma is part of a global disorganization of all processes that have their origin in the central nervous system. These include motor ability, sensation, cognition, and language. Specific disruptions of the language receptive and expressive processes include qualities of inappropriateness, fragmentation, tangentiality, irrelevancy, sparsity, and disinhibition. Any of these pathologic qualities may be present to a certain degree and may persist for indeterminate periods of time.

Patients may exhibit a rather striking deficit in associative language. Levin (1982) terms this deficit "conceptual disorganization," from 1 of the 18 rating scales on the Brief Psychiatric Rating Scale (Overall and Gorham, 1962). Levin includes conceptual disorganization as a psychiatric consequence of closed head injury. Whether psychiatric or linguistic, this symptom has not been adequately defined or followed in long term studies. Patients with this disturbance associate freely to a statement, bringing in many extraneous elements. The associations usually follow from each other, but often deviate far from the topic of conversation. All aspects of a problem may be addressed, but the central issue is not stated or is buried in extraneous associations.

Associations are often concrete with the abstract meaning ignored. The presence of this symptom is striking. Although this deficit is usually obvious, its presence may be further determined by asking the patient to interpret familiar proverbs. The patient with conceptual disorganization is verbose, concrete, and speaks around the meaning of the proverb, but does not arrive at the correct meaning.

Case Study

C.S. is a 19½ year old black female who sustained severe closed head injury as a pedestrian at age 16½. Initial CT scan showed fracture to the left petrous bone and right cerebral edema. Intracranial pressure was elevated during the acute course. On the seventh day the patient became more unresponsive and had three episodes of seizure activity. Repeat CT scan showed bifrontal cerebral edema and mild ventricular enlargement. Coma terminated after 19 days. Twenty-nine days after injury the patient was alert but easily distractable. Speech was dysarthric. The patient was disoriented to place and time. She was anomic and perseverative in her answers to questions. Predominant affect was mild agitation. Six months after her injury, the patient was consistently oriented with coherent speech, but thought processes were disordered. Her predominant affect was silly and immature. The patient was interviewed 1 year after her accident. Affect was then serious and concerned. Speech and thought processes were slow. The patient continued to demonstrate disordered associations and impairment of abstract thinking. She stated that a coat and a dress are similar because "Both have material and are open at the bottom, both have sleeves and buttons." The proverb "When the cat's away, the mice will play" was interpreted as "Cats are always after mice, and the mouse feels freedom if he doesn't see a cat real close." The proverb "Don't count your chickens before they are hatched" was interpreted as "If you have a problem, don't celebrate solving it if it hasn't been solved yet." In discussing a topic the patient spoke in a verbose manner, associating from one loosely connected idea to another, but often missing the central idea.

Neuropsychologic deficits are more common with increasing severity of injury. Their presence is extremely important in the determination of the posttraumatic functional outcome. These symptoms influence cognitive abilities and psychiatric status as well. A patient with full motor recovery and restored intelligence may remain mentally handicapped if burdened with prominent neuropsychologic deficits. These deficits also lend an air of peculiarity to the person recovering from severe head injury. As soon as they are viewed as different or strange, patients are often singled out and ostracized from peer groups. Increasing social isolation becomes a contributing factor to the formation of reactive psychiatric disturbances. Patients who have disturbances that are especially prominent in social interaction are most affected. Such symptoms include pronounced slowness of speech and thought processes, a prominent staring expression, aversion of gaze, and conceptual disorganization.

Neuropsychologic testing in children and adolescents after severe closed head injury has yielded a pattern of deficits similar to that seen in the adult population. In addition to memory impairment, deficits are seen in speed of motor performance, visuospatial functioning and somatosensory abilities. Although these deficits are common, they may differ in severity of each in any one individual. In one neuropsychologic outcome study (Levin and Eisenberg, 1979), at least one third of the patients were impaired in each major area of deficit studied (language, visuospatial, memory, somatosensory, motor speed).

NEUROPSYCHOLOGIC PROBLEMS

Certain neuropsychologic deficits are frequently observed in testing performed at various times after injury. Various types of memory loss include short term, long term, retrieval, and storage components. In one 10 year follow-up study, nearly 25 percent of the head injured child population continued to manifest verbal memory deficits (Gaidolfi and Vignolo, 1980). Persistent memory loss contributes significantly to disability, and memory deficits seriously impede academic, vocational, and social interactions. Students may be unable to remember material from lectures or a homework assignment. Employees may find it difficult to remember sequences in the performance of a job assignment. A social relationship may be disrupted when an important promise is not remembered.

Case History

C.E. is a 23 year old white male who suffered closed head injury as a passenger at age 19. Initial CT scan revealed diffuse cerebral swelling. The patient was comatose for 5 days. C.E. demonstrated deficits in rote sequential auditory memory skills at the completion of a 2 month rehabilitation program. He performed at the first grade level on a test requiring literal recall and inferential reasoning about orally presented stories. After discharge, the patient sought employment in retail sales. Being likable and sociable, the patient obtained employment easily. Once employed, C.E. experienced difficulty in remembering schedules, locations of items, and instructions from his supervisor. He has lost several jobs on this account.

Slowness of motor speed, reaction time, speech, and thought is another other deficit that persists. Patients often describe slowed thinking. Decreased speed of information processing has been demonstrated in adult patients (Gronwall and Sampson, 1974). Such slowness hinders verbal and written performance. Students are unable to copy classroom assignments at the speed necessary to keep up with the class. They are reluctant to speak because a single sentence may take two or three times longer to say. This reluctance extends to social conversations as well, since individuals risk being cut off or ignored by people who are unsympathetic or impatient.

Visuoperceptual and *somatosensory deficits* may persist and lead to disability. The long term recovery of these functions has not been examined. Deficits have been noted on such tests as finger localization, visuospatial functioning, and graphesthesia. Visuoperceptual function refers to a person's visual interpretation of shapes, sizes, distances, and locations of objects in the environment. The Bender Gestalt Test, for example, evaluates visuoperceptual ability in the copying of nine geometric figures. Deviations from the presented figures demonstrate visuoperceptual deficits. Somatosensory function refers to abilities of the sensory organs to assist in definition and localization of input. A test of graphesthetic ability may be used to evaluate somatosensory function. While the patient's eyes are closed, the examiner traces numbers onto the patient's palm. The patient is asked to indicate the correct number. Failure to give the correct number is an indication of loss of graphesthetic ability.

Hearing and balance are mediated by a common set of structures in the central nervous system. Significant damage to any of these structures in the brainstem, cerebellum, or cortex leads to *hearing loss or vertigo,* a disturbance of position regulation which results in dizziness and impaired balance. A thorough otologic and audiologic evaluation is performed as part of a rehabilitation assessment. Many symptoms of auditory and vestibular malfunction are persistent, including some types of sensorineural hearing loss (Healy, 1982).

Defects of smell have been documented in 72 of 1,000 adults with severe head injury (Leigh, 1943). In 12 of these cases, there was a perversion of smell perception, termed parosmia. Recovery of olfactory function was noted in 6 of the 72 cases and was usually seen within 6 months of the injury.

It is likely that deficits in various somatosensory functions of vision, touch, smell, and hearing combine with deficits in memory to result in a pervasive disturbance of *perception.* This disturbance may result in a patient's not being sure of where he is and how to proceed from his present location. A disturbance in auditory perception may result in poor comprehension of what others are saying or a misreading of auditory social cues in conversation.

Neurologic deficits tend to persist, but they do not appear to impede heavily on functions of walking and self-care. Brink and colleagues (1980) described 344 patients under 18 years of age, with a median coma duration of 5 to 6 weeks. Only 10 percent of the study population had a normal neurologic exam one year after injury. Thirty-eight percent of the population were spastic, 8 percent were ataxic, and 39 percent were both spastic and ataxic, yet 73 percent were independent in ambulation and self-care skills 1 year after their injury. In Richardson's follow-up (1963) of 10 patients at least 2 years after injury, 7 of the patients had prominent neurologic sequelae, including hemiparesis, hemiplegia, and involuntary movements. He noted that neurologic improvement continued over 3 years, in some cases.

Klonoff and coworkers (1977) found neurologic abnormalities least likely to show change over the 5 year follow-up period. At the completion of the 5 year period, 38 percent of those injured when they were younger than 9 years old and 31 percent of those injured when they were older than 9 years showed persistent neurologic deficits.

Enlargement of the ventricles of the brain is a common event after severe head trauma. The ventricles are cavities inside the brain which form a system of passage for the cerebrospinal fluid (CSF) that circulates over and inside the brain. The spinal fluid serves as a protective cushion and as a carrier of nutrients and wastes back and forth from the blood. Within weeks after severe injury, enlargement of part or all of the ventricular system has been noted in from 40 to 78 percent of different CT scan investigations (Levin, 1981). Enlargement of the ventricles may indicate an obstruction to the flow of CSF such as may result from a posttraumatic subarachnoid hemorrhage. This possibility can be investigated by a radiologic procedure such as isotope cisternography. If the ventricular dilation is due to an obstruction, then the dilatation is reversible with the relief of the obstruction by a surgical procedure. The CSF can be shunted from the obstructed ventricular system by placement of a tube from the ventricular system to a blood vessel to provide an exit for the built-up fluid.

This complication of posttraumatic communicating hydrocephalus is relatively uncommon, with an estimated frequency of 1 to 2 percent of patients admitted for a head injury (Granholm and Srendgaard, 1972). The efficacy of the CSF shunting procedure for this complication has not been adequately evaluated.

More commonly, the ventricular enlargement is an indication of diffuse loss of cerebral substance. The enlargement may be diffuse and symmetrical, involving the entire ventricular system, or the enlargement may be a focal dilatation of part of a ventricle on only one side. The temporal lobe is particularly vulnerable to injury in blunt trauma and focal dilatation of the temporal horn of the lateral ventricle may occur. Focal neurologic signs or symptoms have been associated with this dilatation of the temporal horn (Lewin, 1965; Potter, 1970). This increase in ventricular size has been studied by use of encephalography and more recently by CT scan procedures. Hawkins (1976) found a relationship between ventricular size and residual functional disability in 96 head injured patients and 56 matched controls. The follow-up period was variable in this retrospective study. Other studies have found an association between enlarged ventricles and residual neurologic impairment and between enlarged ventricles and social and vocational impairment. Levin (1981) studied neuropsychologic function at least 6 months after injury in 32 young adults who had suffered closed head injury. Neuropsychologic function was also tested in 32 age matched controls. Twenty-three or 72 percent of the study population showed evidence of increased ventricular volume in comparison with control values. Within the control group, the ventricular volume of older controls exceeded that of younger controls and ventricular volume of symptomatic non–brain damaged patients exceeded that of the normal patients. A quarter of the patients with increased ventricular volumes also showed evidence of widening of the cerebral sulci, another sign of cortical atrophy. Levin's evaluation included the Wechsler Adult Intelligence Scale (WAIS), assessment of verbal learning and memory, and continuous recognition memory of line drawings. The study found a relationship between ventricular enlargement and both duration of coma and persistence of cognitive deficits measured by the neuropsychologic battery. Evidence of deficits included a Wechsler scale below 85, impaired learning and retention of a word list, and impaired continuous recognition memory.

Although in most circumstances the neurologic deficit is not severe or strategic enough to impede walking and self-care, it is probable that it contributes to the creation and intensity of the *psychologic sequelae* that arise. Spasticity and movement disorders, including ataxia, result in limitation of movement and in physical disfigurement. Both deficits tend to have negative effects on body image, which in turn contribute to a damaged self-concept. Preoccupation with the body and its development forms an integral component of maturation in developing adolescents. If there is a generalized slowdown of motion, patients have difficulty keeping up with the activities of peers. A movement disorder may affect balance or may result in an involuntary movement that impairs function and brings attention to the patient.

Children react differently to their handicaps. Many patients exhibit initial stress and then gradually accept the handicap while learning to cope under the changed conditions. Some patients become withdrawn and depressed and shun others.

A less adaptive reaction is a denial of the handicap's existence. Such a reaction occurred in a 14 year old male adolescent.

Case History

J.C. is a $16\frac{10}{12}$ year old white male who suffered severe closed head injury at age $13\frac{7}{12}$ when his bicycle was hit by a truck. The patient remained comatose for 5 days. CT scans were negative for focal lesions. Three months after injury, the patient had a persistent paralysis of his left upper extremity and a healing fracture of his right knee.

Neuropsychologic deficits included impaired memory, language comprehension, and visual perceptual skills.

The patient had been an average student, completing eight grades at a parochial school. He had been well adjusted without major emotional or behavior problems. J.C.'s 14 year old brother, to whom he had been very close, had been murdered when J.C. was 8.

The patient's neuropsychologic deficits lessened over the next 2 years. His language skills returned to normal levels. The patient demonstrated obvious physical disability. He maintained a persistent staring expression. The knee fracture had affected the growth plate, resulting in a 1 inch leg-length discrepancy. His paralyzed left arm was small and remained flexed at the elbow. As if attempting to hide the disfigurement, the patient wore a baseball mitt on the hand and throughout the interview threw a ball into the mitt. When asked, he stated that his left arm was not as strong as his right arm, but was almost as strong.

After hospital discharge, the patient developed a behavior disorder that gradually worsened. He frequently displayed anger in an impulsive fashion. He became verbally and physically aggressive to his mother. He displayed poor motivation in regard to his school work. He showed poor judgment in choosing predelinquent younger boys as companions. The patient denied the existence of his misbehavior and the presence of physical disability.

The family was referred for treatment to the division of behavioral psychology. Over a 6 month period, J.C. and his parents worked on methods to develop open communication and to develop problem-solving techniques. The family worked together on conflict-resolution training methods. After several sessions, they were able to use these steps to resolve specific problems. By the end of the treatment period J.C.'s home behavior and attitude had improved. The parents also made positive adjustments in their lives and reported overall improved family functioning.

Paralysis is an uncommon sequela of severe closed head injury. In the Rancho Los Amigos series of 52 patients, only 3 patients who regained consciousness were unable to walk (Brink et al., 1970). Two patients were quadriplegic with ataxia and one patient had a concomitant spinal cord injury with paraplegia.

Simultaneous head and spinal cord injuries are unusual. The National Head and Spinal Cord Injury survey sample of 1974 found 1,236 head and/or spinal cord injuries, of which 1,210 were head injuries and 31 were spinal cord injuries (Kalsbeek, 1980).

A small number of head injured children and adolescents are left with very severe physical and/or mental handicaps. These patients are often multiply handicapped and are the most severely impaired group reentering the school. Paralysis of limbs may be combined with tracheostomy dependency, ventilator dependency, aphonia, or gastrostomy dependency. Such extreme physical incapacity is often combined with varying degrees of neuropsychologic and psychiatric impairment.

Impaired swallowing is often a temporary condition following severe closed head injury. The act of normal swallowing is a complicated neuromuscular event, involving the coordination of multiple peripheral and central nervous system components and their muscle connections. A swallowing center located within the medullary part of the brainstem has a role in the control and organization of the entire action. In most circumstances the swallowing impairment resolves during the period of early recovery.

Aspiration is the most dreaded complication of an impaired swallowing mechanism. Food material, either solid or liquid, enters the respiratory tract instead of following the regular course through the digestive tract. This abnormal passage of food material may lead to a catastrophe by completely obstructing the trachea and cutting off the air supply to the lungs. Such complete obstruction, if not quickly relieved, leads to death. Lesser degrees of aspiration are much more common and may escape detection. Small quantities of the solid or liquid meal enter the respiratory tract due to the poor coordination of the swallowing process. The presence of such foreign substances is irritating to the respiratory tract; it responds with an inflammation called chemical or aspiration pneumonia. If bacteria enter the trachea along with the food, bacterial pneumonia or a lung abscess may result.

Other symptoms that lead to consideration of a swallowing disorder include nasal regurgitation of food and the presence of heartburn (Morrell, 1984).

Rehabilitation specialists are aware of these swallowing disorders and their frequency during the early recovery process. The Kennedy Institute has assembled a feeding team to evaluate and treat patients, since resumption of oral feeding is usually attempted after intensive care. Although the team has representation from nine specialty areas, primary responsibility resides in a smaller group consisting of the nurse, the nutritionist, the occupational therapist, and the speech and language pathologist. Patients are observed and closely supervised at all mealtimes.

When *dysphagia*, or impaired swallowing, is subtle or questionable, specialists such as neurologists and radiologists perform examinations and radiologic procedures. By the time of hospital discharge, usually 3 to 6 months after injury, most patients are able to eat with minimal assistance. Prolonged dysphagia is a severe complication and is usually present with other evidences of severe disability. This complication requires cessation of all oral feedings and the use of a nasogastric tube or a gastrostomy for feeding. Spontaneous improvement may result after prolonged dysphagia, but the natural history of this disorder is unknown. Many innovative treatment strategies are currently being devised and tested by carefully constructed feeding protocols. Occasionally surgical intervention is necessary, either to improve the chances of swallowing and protecting the airway or to provide an alternative route by which the patient can receive food and water (Miller and Groher, 1984).

The resumption of oral feeding is an event of great psychological importance to families. Eating is a primary function invested with connotations of health, strength, and independence. The first attempts at oral feeding may be made before the patient is at the level of simple commands. In most cases, as the patient emerges from coma, the swallowing function gradually improves. Most patients also assume increasing responsibility for the events surrounding feeding: obtaining the food, preparing it, and observing a reasonable degree of etiquette. When such a sequence does not occur, the results may be devastating for parents.

Patients fed by gastrostomy do not participate in normal family meals. The feeding itself is a mechanical procedure often without pleasurable social interaction. At times feeding is carried out by a non-family member such as a licensed practical nurse. The patient forfeits social interaction at the family table and the customary holiday celebrations centered around food. For these reasons persistent dysphagia may be more difficult to accept than other forms of handicap. Little information is available concerning the personal reaction of patients. In most instances where the patient is depressed or anxious, dysphagia is just one of multiple handicaps to which the patient is responding. The family response may be a peculiar type of denial that follows a certain pattern. Parents are informed of the probable persistence of dysphagia during the rehabilitation course of their child, and the clinical and radiologic evidence is carefully explained. When the parents are instructed to avoid all oral feedings, they do not contest the findings or recommendations. When they are alone with the child, however, they attempt oral feedings which they do not bring to the attention of staff. Once the child leaves the hospital these parents resume degrees of oral feeding at home, often attempting to get the support of unknowledgeable physicians. Even when there is clear evidence that food is being abnormally diverted into the respiratory tract, these parents will not desist in their efforts. The power of psychologic denial has been illustrated by a case in which a physician anesthesiologist persisted in the oral feeding of her dysphagic son.

Persistent vegetative state, the worst outcome of severe closed head injury, is a condition of unresponsiveness. It is important to distinguish the 5 percent of patients in this condition from those who are severely disabled. In one series of 110 patients with persistent vegetative state, more than one third of the cases were due to trauma, with other causes being stroke, brain tumors, and central nervous system infections (Higashi et al., 1977).

Vegetative patients may have regular periods of sleep and wakefulness with eye opening. Motor responses are abnormal in all extremities. Other behavioral responses exhibited by these patients are response to painful stimuli, eye–following movements, and emotional expressions such as meaningless laughter or weeping. The EEG findings may not correlate with the severity of the injury because normal EEG activity is sometimes demonstrated (Higashi et al., 1977). There is no evidence of mental functioning. Patients destined to recover from coma most often do not exhibit these characteristic signs and symptoms (Jennett and Plum, 1972).

In most cases a persistent vegetative state can be predicted within 3 months of injury. In a series of 94 patients from Glasgow, only 10 percent of the patients regarded as vegetative at 3 months regained consciousness and all of this group remained totally dependent (Jennett and Teasdale, 1981). In a series of 110 patients from Japan, 3 patients regained ability to communicate as social beings; however, only one of these patients regained nearly normal brain function. The mortality rate was 65 percent for the total 3 year period of follow-up.

Occasionally case reports describe remarkable recovery from coma after a very long period of time (Tanhehco and Kaplan, 1982). In one report, a woman comatose for 6 years opened her eyes and became responsive to the environment. After 6 months of rehabilitation, the woman obtained a 12th grade score on the Adult Basic Learning Examination, a subtest of speech and language function.

Existence in a vegetative state is viewed by many as an existence worse than death, or as equivalent to death temporarily postponed (Jennett and Teasdale, 1981). The emotional and economic stresses are very great for families who are involved with a close relative in a vegetative state. Many families remain actively engaged in the day-to-day nursing care of their relative. Some families maintain persistent hope for eventual recovery, although the chances of such an event are negligible. In addition, the continued existence of their relative does not allow for a natural unfolding of the mourning process.

New rehabilitation methods aim to increase the number of patients who emerge from the comatose state. Coma arousal therapy is one such method currently being studied by a collaborative group of researchers in Australia (Miller, 1985). This method involves a battery of noninvasive, atraumatic, sensory stimuli beginning soon after the period of critical care and requiring substantial family involvement. Any conclusion about the efficacy of this method awaits completion and analysis of the controlled study.

PSYCHIATRIC IMPAIRMENT

As patients emerge from coma, they may be deficient in physical and mental capacities. Delirium is the diagnostic term used by psychiatrists to describe this early behavioral cognitive picture. It consists of a number of symptoms that comprise the pervasive early impairment. The first criterion, clouding of consciousness, and the third criterion, disorientation, suggest the period of time which is similar in extent to the posttraumatic amnesia. There is much fluctuation in intensity of these symptoms.

The psychiatric disorders that follow severe head injury consist of the same spectrum of disorders that afflict the non–head injured population. In addition, certain psychiatric disorders stem more directly from the neurologic insult and have prominent neurologic characteristics. These disorders with presumed anatomic or neurologic etiologies are termed organic disorders to distinguish them from those disorders with presumed psychologic or nonneurologic etiologies, which are termed functional disorders. The organic/nonorganic distinction blurs in the case of posttraumatic psychiatric disorders. Memory and somatosensory impairment strongly affect psychiatric disorders such as depression or anxiety and lend an aspect of strangeness or peculiarity to these disorders. For example, head injured patients may demonstrate great emotional lability. With little provocation patients may change from a state of happiness to a state of depression over an interval of seconds. During the period of depression, a patient might impulsively make a suicide gesture that is later disowned or forgotten when the affect switches back to a more positive one. These qualities of lability, impulsivity, and forgetfulness are characteristics that stem from brain injury and that influence the form that the symptom of depression assumes. Many of these symptoms are characteristic of brain damage in general and many may be seen in a noninjured population. Sometimes these symptoms may be found in combination with other types of posttraumatic deficits that will in turn color the clinical picture.

Many of the children and adolescents who suffer severe closed head injury have a history of premorbid social and academic maladjustment. In a Kennedy Institute sample, 46 percent of the school aged population had premorbid academic problems. Many of the younger children had a history of attentional problems and hyperactivity, other behavior problems and learning disabilities. Many of the older children and teenagers had exhibited antisocial behaviors and had experimented with or abused alcohol and drugs. The percentage of driver fatalities with measurable blood alcohol levels rises with increasing age, from 40 percent at age 16 to 63 percent at age 19 (Fell, 1982). In a follow-up study of adults with severe head injuries, 46 percent of the patient population had a history of premorbid psychiatric symptoms consisting of chronic neurotic symptoms, heavy drinking, petty crime, low intelligence, and chronic schizophrenia (Fahy, Irving, and Millac, 1967).

The relationship among the premorbid psychiatric status, the early posttraumatic sequelae, and the late posttraumatic sequelae remains to be clarified. In adult patients with negative premorbid psychiatric histories, agitated behavior in the early posttraumatic period was predictive of late posttraumatic psychiatric sequelae—excessive anxiety and depression, greater thinking disturbance, and generally increased psychopathology (Levin and Grossman, 1978).

Children and adolescents with premorbid psychiatric problems are at increased risk for the development of early and late posttraumatic psychiatric sequelae. The symptom may be different or the same or an accentuated form of the same premorbid symptom. The symptom may begin early after emergence from coma or later after termination of the PTA. The duration and intensity of the symptom will vary. The Kennedy patient T.H. (discussed on p. 19) with a pronounced history of premorbid aggression developed a severe posttraumatic aggressive disorder 4 days after emergence from coma while still in posttraumatic amnesia.

Delirium best describes, from a psychiatric point of view, the period of coma and emergence from coma. The Diagnostic and Statistical Manual III (DSM III) states that the duration of delirium is brief and rarely persists longer than a month. Many head trauma patients traverse several weeks of coma followed by a long period of emergence from coma during which they fulfill the diagnostic criteria for delirium. The condition is treated by creating an environment for the patient that is nonstimulating yet orienting. Because the patient's mental processes are disorganized and his or her capacity to focus and sustain attention is very limited, the staff works to keep contacts limited and simple in content. Reminders such as a family picture and a clock serve to orient repeatedly the patient with impaired memory and visuospatial ability.

Perceptual disturbances such as hallucinations are common during delirium. These may become sources of great fear or agitation to patients.

Dementia is diagnosed when the patient continues to show global cognitive, language, and personality impairment to a degree that interferes with social and academic functioning. The necessary criteria for the diagnosis are intellectual and memory impairment. Personality change may be present.

Amnestic syndrome is another psychiatric diagnosis that describes a deficit of short and long term memory. Four other diagnoses—organic delusional syndrome, organic hallucinosis, organic affective syndrome, and organic personality syndrome— are specific psychiatric derangements that may occur after the termination of delirium. All of these organic mental disorders may persist or may end after a length of time, with or without intervention.

Physical and *cognitive/language impairment* tends to lessen during the first year after injury while psychiatric impairment tends to emerge during the first year after injury. Children and adolescents with premorbid psychiatric problems are at increased risk for the development of posttraumatic psychiatric problems. However, even those children without premorbid psychiatric problems are at increased risk. In a controlled prospective study of 31 children with severe head injuries (Brown, Chadwick, Shaffer, Rutter, and Traub, 1981), half of the children without premorbid problems had developed psychiatric problems within a year, while all of the study population with mild premorbid problems demonstrated psychiatric problems within this time.

Rutter (1981) also describes other contributing factors to psychiatric disorders. The severity of injury increases risk for development of psychiatric disorder, but severity of injury does not show the same positive relationship that it does to cognitive impairment. The degree of cognitive impairment shows some relation to psychiatric disorder as does also the presence of a seizure disorder or an abnormal EEG. Poor family functioning is another risk factor. Rutter defined impaired family functioning by criteria including psychiatric disorder in mother or father, unhappy marriage, and four or more siblings.

Rutter concludes from his studies of posttraumatic psychiatric problems in children that most children with psychiatric disorders show the usual mixture of emotional and conduct disorders found in children without brain damage and that there is no specific posttraumatic psychiatric syndrome except social disinhibition. Head injured children differ from non–head injured control subjects in a greater number of most types of symptoms.

DSM III—Diagnostic and Statistical Manual of Mental Disorders: A diagnostic manual of behavioral and psychiatric disorders as currently understood. Criteria for diagnosis are listed for all entries. Representative diagnostic chapters are entitled anxiety disorders, substance use disorders, and affective disorders. One chapter is devoted to organic mental disorders. Another describes diagnoses seen in infancy, childhood, and adolescence. This manual is currently used in all accredited psychiatric facilities as well as by many other mental health professionals.

Pica and hyperphagia are behaviors that often begin soon after the patient emerges from coma. Pica refers to the ingestion of substances not ordinarily classified as food. Many ingested objects are toxic and themselves lead to illness (e.g., the ingestion of paint chips leading to lead poisoning). Hyperphagia refers to voracious food-seeking and overeating that may result in prominent weight gain. These two behaviors may occur together or apart. They usually abate after termination of the posttraumatic amnesia. If hyperphagia persists, behavioral management is usually attempted in order to control the food-seeking behavior. No medication has yet been found helpful. Some observers view these behaviors as evidence of temporary endocrine dysfunction. Since regulation of appetite and satiety resides in the posterior hypothalamus, disruption of this structure may lead to indiscriminate eating behavior. Other observers view hyperphagia and pica as an indication of a generalized process of disinhibition, manifested by other symptoms as well. Endocrine, blood, and urine studies on a series of posttraumatic patients would be helpful in clarifying the role of the endocrine organs in these disorders. A confounding factor to the symptom of hyperphagia is the use of psychotropic medications, notably haloperidol, chlorpromazine, and thioridazine to control agitated behavior. These medications may also result in hyperphagic behavior, and their use may have be curtailed for this reason.

> Disinhibition: Exhibition of behaviors that show poor self-regulation of words and actions. It is assumed that the neural regulation over what is said or done is temporarily or permanently damaged.

Agitation, hyperactivity and *aggression* are three posttraumatic motoric behavioral symptoms. The term "agitation" is usually confined to the early posttraumatic behavior after emergence from coma and has been described in the first chapter.

When motor restlessness persists beyond the termination of the PTA, it is usually called hyperactivity. High degrees of motor activity usually abate during subsequent months. In cases of persistent hyperactivity, the posttraumatic symptom may be an exacerbation of a premorbid symptom. The DSM III diagnosis of Attention Deficit Disorder with Hyperactivity is made if the other two diagnostic criteria of this syndrome, inattention and impulsivity, are also fulfilled. The treatment of hyperactivity is behavioral, with an emphasis on consistent and structured management. If the diagnosis of Attention Deficit Disorder is made, then a treatment trial with psychostimulants is often made. No controlled studies have been published on the use of medication in the treatment of posttraumatic hyperactivity disorders.

Behavior may become aggressive at any time following emergence from coma. Early aggression appears indiscriminate in its focus and is indistinguishable from agitation. After termination of the posttraumatic amnesia, aggressive behavior often becomes more focused, occurring when the patient is stressed or provoked. In one patient, early hyperphagia changed in its character to an aggressive food-seeking behavior. After several months the hyperphagia abated, but the aggression persisted and became more severe. Often the aggression will be impulsive and explosive. At these times the DSM III behavioral diagnosis of Intermittent Explosive Disorder may be made. Impulsive and explosive behaviors cause great tension in families.

The treatment of posttraumatic aggression is as difficult as the treatment of other types of aggression. Behavior treatments that utilize methods of conditioning have had some success.

A number of medications have been tried and anecdotal reports of success of one or the other have been published. These medications include propranolol, lithium, and diazepam. Occasionally the severity of aggression requires psychiatric hospitalization. The most common hospital therapy is a combination of a closely structured milieu and the use of psychotropic medications. The psychotropic medications used most commonly, haloperidol and chlorpromazine, lack a specific activity against aggression. They sedate the patient and decrease levels of motor activity. Their use must be monitored carefully, as oversedation and pronounced motor side effects may occur.

Lability and *impulsivity* are posttraumatic behaviors that are common following a variety of brain dysfunctions. Lability refers to an instability of affect. It is an old, still widely used term which has been dropped from the DSM III. The clinical presentation is often striking. A person with labile affect switches unpredictably from one emotional state to another—discussing a factual issue in a neutral manner one minute, then suddenly becoming sad and tearful, for example. Often nothing in the content of the conversation suggests a change in emotional state; in fact, the change in emotion is often inappropriate. Companions often respond in an angry fashion, thinking the sudden change in affect was intentional and blaming the patient for being disruptive. The patient is often perplexed, not understanding the origin of the sadness. Lability is most prominent in early recovery but may be persistent.

Impulsivity is most often described as a late appearing psychiatric behavior that tends to persist. It shares with lability the essential characteristics of suddeness and unpredictability. The concern here is with impulsive actions that are maladaptive, such as disruptive violent or aggressive actions. Labile behavior is attributed to nervous system impairment, but the term impulsive behavior carries the connotation that the behavior is under some degree of volitional control. An essential feature of disorders of impulse control, as defined by the DSM III, is the experiencing of pleasure, gratification, or release at the time of the impulsive act. The act is considered to be consonant with the immediate conscious wish of the individual.

No medical or psychologic treatment has been found to influence the symptom of lability. Patients and family members may need to be educated about labile behavior, its meaning, and its cause. Hopefully, occurrences can be diminished in importance and not result in social upsets. Treatment of impulse disorders poses a much more serious problem. These disorders may lead to grossly impaired social relationships, depending on the frequency and intensity of the outbursts. Psychologic and drug therapies have not been beneficial. The possibility of a seizure disorder should be investigated, as temporal lobe epilepsy may be characterized by explosive violent outbursts. Antiseizure medication is sometimes used in this circumstance. If a patient's symptomatology poses danger to self or others, then hospitalization is necessary. When destructive violent acts are carried out, the patient may be jailed. In the case of intermittent explosive disorders, males are likely to be placed in a correctional institution and females in a mental health facility (American Psychiatric Association, 1980).

Apathy, the loss of drive or motivation, is attributed to frontal lobe damage. Extreme degrees of apathy often dominate the posttraumatic personality and result in great functional disability. Apathy is more likely to be socially accepted if it coexists with other physical or mental handicaps. Occasionally a patient may have no other physical or mental deficits, yet remain functionless. If left unattended, the patient spends waking hours sitting, appears content but is unmotivated, and moves only to attend to bodily functions. Such patients may listen to music or watch television, but do not object if these sources of stimulation are removed. Milder degrees of apathy result in less incapacity but still figure as maladaptive traits. Lack of motivation is particularly striking in a previously well-motivated individual. A tendency exists for persons close to the patient to assign purposeful intent to such exasperating passivity.

No psychiatric or medical treatment will restore or increase a person's drive. It is important that family members understand this symptom and do not attribute it to laziness. It would be possible for a patient to resume school or employment were it not for this lack of drive. A family member often assumes the burden of directing the patient's day. Once at school or work, the patient accepts and cooperates with the structured routine until it is time to return home. After being urged to complete homework assignments, the patient is then free to sit the rest of the evening. The patient voices little objection to this routine, simply lacking the motivation to resist. The motivating force comes from the outside and the venture's success depends on a family member's willingness to take on this great responsibility. Reduced drive is less noticeable in childhood because a young child's activities are usually under the direction of a responsible adult. Even if a child is described as unmotivated, this behavior is not as troublesome as it is in an adult, who is expected to function independently.

There may be positive aspects to a reduction in drive. Patients with premorbid personality traits of hostility, aggressiveness, and suspiciousness may lose these traits. Under these uncommon circumstances, some families will report improved personality functioning of their brain injured member. The resultant affect or emotional state is described sometimes as shallow or bland.

Inattention and *impaired concentration* are two behavioral symptoms that figure prominently in childhood, as they frequently result in impaired school performance. Inattention is a necessary criterion of the delirious state that may occur after emergence from coma. The DSM III describes it as a reduced capacity to focus and sustain attention to environmental stimuli. The patient rapidly shifts focus from one object or event to another, or may be described as easily distractible. Impaired concentration refers to a person's inability to attend and contemplate a particular stimulus with any depth and for any length of time. In the early stages of treatment, inattention is viewed as having a neurologic cause. As the delirious state subsides, inattention may abate somewhat, but still persists to a lesser degree. If a child shows symptoms of impulsivity and hyperactivity in addition to inattention, and if the injury occurred before age 7, then the diagnostic criteria for Attention Deficit Disorder with Hyperactivity are met. Symptoms of inattention necessary for the diagnosis are three of the following: The child (1) often fails to finish things; (2) often doesn't seem to listen; (3) is easily distracted; and (4) has difficulty concentrating on school work or other tasks requiring sustained attention. If the child is inattentive and impulsive but lacks hyperactivity, Attention Deficit Disorder without Hyperactivity is the diagnosis. The diagnosis may be made in an older patient by retrospective fulfillment of criteria during childhood and is called Attention Deficit Disorder, Residual Type.

The posttraumatic attentional problem can be an exacerbation of a preexisting symptom. Many of the patients with prominent posttraumatic inattention have a documented history of premorbid inattention. Inattention is missing, however, in the premorbid history of others who develop the symptom after injury. Early inattention is treated as part of the delirious state. The patient is cared for in a protective, orienting environment. Medication is used only if patients remain dangerous to themselves or others. If inattention, impaired concentration, or easy distractibility are isolated problems, they are addressed with the use of structured environments and close educational or social supervision. Cognitive rehabilitation adult programs have focused on attentional deficits since they often lead to impaired work performance. Tasks have been devised in these programs to focus specifically on improvement of attention. Computer software programs designed to improve academic performance have been adapted for study strategies that improve attention and concentration.

Certain behaviors appear indicative of central nervous system disinhibition. Researchers theorize that certain processes are controlled or held in check by inhibitory factors, namely systems of inhibitory neurons in the nervous system. This notion is supported by the existence of specific neurotransmitters and neuronal systems whose main function is to inhibit the activity of other neuronal systems. At this time it is possible only to speculate that one or more neuronal systems responsible for inhibiting certain behaviors has been damaged by head trauma when disinhibition is present.

Rutter (1981) categorizes the following behaviors as disinhibited: marked outspokenness, undressing in public, making very personal remarks, asking embarrassing questions, impulsiveness, overtalkativeness, and forgetfulness. He observed that this group of behaviors distinguished a head injured population from a control group of children with orthopedic injuries. Rutter noted the similarity of these behaviors to those described as the frontal lobe syndrome in adults with focal brain damage

(Lishman, 1968). Frontal lobe damage or disinhibition has been implicated in the etiology of these socially inappropriate behaviors seen in children and adolescents.

The clinical picture of these behaviors is often striking and quite often disturbing to the unknowledgeable. The patient appears impaired in his ability to make a good judgment in social circumstances. Parents are disturbed when a previously polite teenage son sprinkles his conversation with obscenities. Parents are also disturbed when a 10 year old girl shows physical familiarity with casual acquaintances. The behavior of disinhibited children and adolescents is equally disturbing to their teachers. Fortunately, these behaviors tend to lessen in most patients as recovery proceeds.

Medication has had no role in management of this behavior. Behavior programs, often instituted in collaboration with the school system, have been somewhat successful with a small number of pupils.

Perseveration is another behavior more commonly noted in brain injured patients. Perseveration refers to repetition of words or actions when such repetition is unnecessary or even inappropriate. Perseveration may be a normal phenomenon in a young child who may repeat an amusing statement several times to his audience. Perseveration in a brain injured child may persist from early recovery and is often troublesome. Neither young children nor adolescents appear to be aware of the negative effect that these repetitive requests or actions have on others. Behavior management has been used to treat this symptom.

Psychotic disorders are the most severe type of posttraumatic psychiatric sequelae. In the DSM III the term psychotic indicates a gross impairment in reality testing. These disorders appear with regularity after closed head injury, and may manifest at any time after the patient emerges from coma. These psychoses tend to occur earlier after a diffuse closed head injury followed by a long period of coma than after other types of nervous system injury.

Posttraumatic psychoses occur in a variety of forms. The diagnoses of delirium and dementia are given to the early psychotic disorders, as these states involve a loss of contact with reality. An agitated person who is disoriented and who describes visions is diagnosed as delirious.

Later psychotic behavior may fit a number of diagnoses. Patients can experience an episode of psychosis that occurs once and never recurs, or that occurs a number of times. Late posttraumatic psychoses are either affective or schizophrenic in nature, depending on the predominant symptoms. Affective psychoses fulfill either diagnostic criteria for major affective disorders (mania or depression) or less stringent criteria for organic affective syndrome. An elevated, expansive, depressed, or irritable mood may predominate with alternation in mood states. If a patient alternates between manic and depressive episodes, then a bipolar disorder is present. Symptoms of manic or depressed affect must be present. Psychotic features of delusions or hallucinations must be consistent with the described affect. It is sometimes difficult for caregivers to distinguish a patient with inappropriate silly disinhibited behavior from an overtalkative manic patient with inflated self-esteem.

If thought disorder is the predominant symptom, then the diagnosis fits best into the schizophrenia-like group of psychoses. Making the difficult distinction, however, between a psychotic process and the variety of speech and language disorders that occur following closed head injury is important. Before a diagnosis of psychotic thought disorder is reached, specific criteria must be fulfilled, including deterioration from a previous level of functioning. Posttraumatic psychoses in which thought disorganization predominates include schizophrenic disorders, paranoid disorders, organic hallucinosis, organic delusional syndrome, and brief reactive psychosis. Patients are treated in or out of a hospital according to the severity of their psychoses. When they can be managed by families and are compliant about taking medication, home treatment is preferable. If not, then medications are instituted in the structured setting of a psychiatric ward so that the patient can regain control. Medications used in the treatment of psychotic thinking disorders have not improved the condition of patients suffering from the posttraumatic language disorders referred to as "conceptual disorganization" or "disinhibited language."

In the following history, the patient's predominant symptom changed from disordered thinking to disordered affect as the pattern of chronic psychosis evolved.

Case History

C.E. was a $19\frac{9}{12}$ year old white adolescent male when he suffered severe closed head injury as a passenger. He had been
drinking with the driver earlier in the evening. CT scan showed
diffuse cerebral swelling. The patient was comatose for 5 days
and remained mute for 30 days. C.E. was the fifth of six children.
His parents were divorced. His father was an alcoholic and there
was a history of alcoholism on both sides of the family. There
was no family history of mental illness. C.E. had a history of good
premorbid social adjustment. He left school after 10th grade. He
had been a fairly good student who showed very little interest
in school. The patient was involved in a second minor auto accident as the driver 8 months after the original trauma. He was
mistakenly accused of being intoxicated and jailed because he
demonstrated residual ataxia and dysarthria from the original
accident. Subsequent to this accident the patient became agitated,
delusional, and unable to sleep. He believed that a friend called
up a radio station and requested that the station broadcast static
to the patient. He maintained that dangerous things were coming out of the ceiling vents. The patient was admitted to a psychiatric hospital for treatment of hallucinations, delusions, and
a thought disorder. The patient fulfilled diagnostic criteria for
schizophrenia and was treated with psychotropic medication,
with relief of symptoms. After discharge he remained at home,
spending his time watching TV and listening to music. Attempts
were made to place him in cognitive and vocational rehabilitation programs. He eventually discontinued medication. Two years
after his injury, C.E. was readmitted with symptoms of irritability, decreased sleep, and fearfulness. Lithium was successfully
used to treat the patient's prominent mood disorder. Two months
later the patient slashed his wrists after a family disagreement,
incurring tendon damage. Readmitted to the hospital, the patient
denied symptoms of depression, but stated that he had been
depressed when he cut his wrists. Lithium was discontinued and
the patient was treated with a psychotropic and an antidepres-
sant. The patient was maintained on medication in an outpatient
clinic. He has had two subsequent admissions for symptom
exacerbations of insomnia, grandiosity, rapid thoughts, and
overtalkativeness.

Nonpsychotic mood disorders are commonly seen in the late
posttraumatic period. Anxiety, euphoria, hypomania, and
depression are among these disorders. Symptoms of anxiety may
arise in connection with increased self-consciousness and concern over performance. Euphoria, an increased sense of well-
being, is probably equivalent to hypomania and is commonly

attributed to frontal lobe injury. Euphoria or hypomania is usually an inappropriate response and may be viewed as a disinhibited mood state.

Depression may occur when patients begin to comprehend the meaning and the implications of their injuries. They may respond with feelings of inadequacy, loss of self-esteem, and self-pity. A pessimistic attitude toward the future may prevail. Such a reaction to injury is maladaptive and leads to further impairment in social or occupational functioning. When patients become depressed early in recovery, it is common to find a history of premorbid depression or substance abuse. Depression reappears as a coping mechanism that has been used in the past under conditions of stress.

These reactive, neurotic varieties of depression often respond well to counseling or psychotherapy, which focuses on the demoralization experienced by the patient and aims toward the development of enhanced self-esteem. Some counselors work with the patient to adapt new strategies for improved social and academic functioning. To educate and involve the family in these endeavors is important, so that members can institute beneficial changes in management and discipline. A family history of affective disorders and substance abuse should be elicited, as such disorders have a hereditary predisposition. Antidepressants may sometimes be combined with psychotherapy for increased effectiveness. Antidepressants may be especially useful if either the patient or close family members have been successfully treated with antidepressants in the past.

Mention should be made of the *post-concussion syndrome*, a behavioral syndrome that follows less severe closed head injury in which periods of coma or posttraumatic amnesia are brief. The most common symptoms of this disorder include headache, vertigo, dizziness, fatigue, and irritability. These individual symptoms are also seen after severe injury, but the frequency and combination of symptoms for post-concussion syndrome are different. This symptom complex is seen often in adults but rarely in children. The cause is predominantly organic. It occurs to some extent in one half of adult patients (Rutherford, Merrett, and McDonald, 1977) and coincides with the persistence of acute neurologic and neuropsychologic abnormalities. Neuropathologists can demonstrate structural brain damage after concussive injuries. Aspects such as a high frequency of industrial accidents, an association with litigation, and a persistence in certain personality types suggest a psychological component in the syndrome's appearance in some individuals.

Behavioral problems are more commonly observed after concussive illnesses in children than in adults. Again, these same behavioral symptoms are seen after severe head injury. Ninety percent of 50 children studied by Dillon and Leopold (1961) had marked behavioral changes after brief periods of unconsciousness (two of the children were unconscious from 1 to 6 days). These changes included aggressiveness, antisocial behavior, sluggishness, and withdrawn behavior. Thirty-seven of the 50 children reported headache and 9 of the 50 children reported dizziness. Black, Jeffries, Blumer, Wellner, and Walker (1969) reported on 105 children who had been unconscious for short periods of time (4 percent more than 24 hours). Headache, the most common posttraumatic problem one year after injury, was seen in 27 percent of the study population. The incidence and severity of headache increased with age. The next three symptoms encountered most frequently were anger control problems (20 percent), hyperkinesis (32 percent), and impaired attention (17 percent).

Headache is an uncommon complaint after severe closed head injury. When it occurs, headache is often a symptom of a developing intracranial hematoma in a patient who remains conscious after injury. The reason for this lack of headache and even the patient's lack of recollection of headache in severe closed head injury patients is unknown. The development of a posttraumatic complication such as an aneurysm, however, may be signaled by a headache. Headache commonly occurs after short periods of unconsciousness and is an important component of the post-concussion syndrome following less severe head injury.

> Hematoma: An abnormal collection of blood that has escaped from the circulatory system because of damage to the blood vessels. Depending on its size and location, a hematoma may press on adjacent organs and compromise their function. If the hematoma is large, the consequent loss of blood from the vessels may result in shock.

> Aneurysm: An expansion or ballooning of a vessel wall because of injury or inherent weakness. An aneurysm may press on adjacent structures and cause symptoms. Or the aneurysm may leak or burst to cause a hemorrhage into adjacent tissues.

Fatigue and *slowness* are commonly observed after severe injury, but these symptoms are often pronounced in early recovery. Initially, recovering children may tire easily and need several rest or sleep periods during the day. Rehabilitation specialists often modify therapeutic contacts to several brief bedside sessions daily rather than a single more lengthy session. Months after trauma, these children may continue to demonstrate easy fatigueability and to need a daily afternoon nap. Slowness in motor, speech, and thought processes may also persist. The symptom of slowness is often upsetting to the patient. Slow speech and thought processes are noticeable and identify an otherwise normal-appearing person as handicapped. The person may take a long while to verbalize a thought, during which time other people may become impatient or annoyed or disinterested. Other listeners may attempt to help patients finish a sentence. Such responses often cause patients to limit their verbal communications and even to isolate themselves in order to avoid communication.

The relationship between severe head injury and *delinquency* is currently being explored. Lewis, Shanok, and Balla (1979) reported that incarcerated delinquents were significantly more likely to have sustained a head or facial injury (62.3 percent) than nonincarcerated delinquents (44.6 percent). This significant difference was evident by age 2. An extensive chart review was the basis of the report. Child abuse was noted more frequently in the medical charts of incarcerated children (10.4 percent) than in the charts of nonincarcerated children (3.6 percent) (Lewis et al., 1979).

More recently, Lewis (1985) has reported on the traits of child delinquents who later committed murder. Psychotic symptomatology and neurologic impairment were the most important individual variables distinguishing the murderers from the ordinary delinquents. Six of the 9 murderers had received head injuries resulting in loss of consciousness.

Other studies of delinquents have documented more frequent head injuries and longer comas among their study populations. Neuropsychologic assessment of delinquent youths has detected wide-spread abnormalities in cognitive, memory, speech, perceptual, and perceptual motor areas. Learning disabilities are also common (Robbins, 1983). Reports have been conflicting in regard to the existence and pattern of deficits, in specific areas such as memory and perceptual motor. However, study populations have varied widely in their makeup according to age, sex percentages, and definition of criminal characteristics: incarcerated versus unincarcerated, adjudicated versus nonadjudicated, violent versus nonviolent.

The role of severe closed head injury in the etiology of delinquent behavior is currently unclear. The high frequency of head injury and loss of consciousness could explain certain neuropsychologic deficits observed in testing. If a significant number of these injuries occurred prior to age 2, then resultant neurologic deficits are expected to be more severe than if the injury occurred after age 2.

The implications of this research focus are important to criminal justice workers. Legal personnel are searching for episodes of abuse and head trauma in the histories of the delinquents they serve. Patients with positive histories are being referred for extensive neuropsychologic evaluations. If deficits are uncovered, lawyers and judges will use the existence of these deficits to seek placement programs that focus on rehabilitation. As the role of head trauma and neuropsychologic deficits in the delinquent process is clarified, then more specific recommendations and treatment strategies for delinquents will evolve.

Outcome is a term used to describe the assessment of a patient's overall ability to function at a certain time after injury. It is a concise statement about the level of independence. Outcome is derived from a profile of deficits, but these deficits are viewed primarily as they impede levels of independence. School adjustment, social relatedness, and leisure time utilization are factors that contribute to outcome. The Glasgow Outcome Scale, for example, is a measure devised by neurosurgeons to evaluate outcome. Patients are divided into four categories: vegetative state, severe disability, moderate disability, and good recovery (Jennett et al., 1976).

Rehabilitation specialists have devised more detailed functional outcome scales in order to follow progress sequentially as therapeutic strategies are carried out. A representative outcome instrument reported from the University of Minnesota is a questionnaire administered to parents of head injured children and young adults. The questionnaire elicits information about gross and fine motor function, cognitive-communication function, social development, and independence (Eiben, 1984). The degree of limitation is further defined as (1) asymptomatic, (2) symptomatic but independent, (3) symptomatic and requiring assistance in a functional area, (4) totally dependent, and (5) deceased.

Outcome measurements of head injured patients reveal that the mental component of disability is most important in determining the level of disability. In the study by Eiben and colleagues (1984), deficits in cognitive function and communication skills contributed proportionately more to disability than did problems in other areas. Functional outcome was less satisfactory in all combined areas than in the individual areas. As with individual deficits, there was a relationship between the coma duration and the eventual functional outcome. Seventy-three percent of 15 patients who were comatose for fewer than 21 days were independent, but 78 percent of 18 patients who were comatose for more than 21 days were dependent.

SUMMARY

Severe closed head injury is a chronic handicapping condition of childhood and adolescence. Once the problems of survival and acute care are resolved, a thorough assessment of resulting deficits is made by a multidisciplinary team of specialists. The more severe the injury and the more protracted the coma, the more likely the occurrence of multiple handicaps. Recovery occurs over a period of months to years and its progress is continually influenced by the concomitant process of development. In the first year after injury, patients exhibit great improvement in physical and cognitive/language deficits. During this year, psychiatric problems appear or reappear and tend to worsen. These psychiatric deficits range from mild to severe in intensity.

The stresses experienced by a family in the acute crisis are great and the recovery is frequently lengthy. The period of chronic handicap may be lifelong. An early evaluation of the family and its coping abilities is valuable to determine where support and extra resources can be placed most effectively. In doing this, health care providers could anticipate certain problems before they occur. The services needed may be multiple and varied and scattered throughout the community. Often a necessary service exists in the community, but a modification may be necessary to serve the specific need of a head injured client. Sometimes even the most sophisticated families are unable to negotiate the system of care. Early in the recovery course, a knowledgeable person such as a case manager or a team of people should undertake the coordination of services among families and various agencies so that the most effective delivery of care can take place.

Most treatment modalities have been adapted from already existing treatments used for similar disorders. As the experience of medical personnel with this population increases, treatment strategies specific for closed head trauma patients will evolve. Examples of this evolution include various techniques of cognitive rehabilitation that focus on modification of maladaptive social behaviors seen after head injury.

Advocacy and support networks provide strength and continuity for all of these rehabilitation endeavors. Because the effort is relatively new (less than 10 years old) definition of available resources and unmet needs is yet to be accomplished in many areas. Organized groups such as state chapters of the National Head Injury Foundation are assuming the leadership in defining needs and services and creating networks for effective care delivery. These groups consist of knowledgeable professionals with a backbone of committed parents and patients.

Chapter **4**

Implications
for School Planning

VARIABILITY

If any quality is most characteristic of the recovery process of
closed head injured students, it is variability. The results of measurement of the effects of head trauma and the descriptions of
such in any one child are elusive in that these effects change
quite rapidly during early recovery. Nowhere is variability the
cause for more difficulty than in school planning.

Prognosis

Variability permeates all dimensions of recovery. While it is possible to generalize about this population and predict some patterns of recovery, the fact that each child will digress in some
way from the general pattern must not be overlooked. This is
a piece of the challenge: *each recovering head injured child is
unique.*

Often the child's rate of change during the first 6 months
after injury is dramatic. Measurable differences can be found
from one day to the next, and sometimes even from morning
to evening. The rapid change tapers off in the ensuing months,
but some change continues for years. Even during this typical

6 month period of great change, recovery will be discouragingly slow, and in some patients there is little change from one week to the next.

Impairment

As might be expected, not all head injuries result in the same damage. The variability of effects of the injury will be influenced by the particular area in which injury occurred (e.g., frontal lobe, brainstem, parietal lobe, and so forth) and the extent of deficits (e.g., mild, moderate or severe; cognitive, language, or motor). Not all parts of the brain recover at the same rate. Thus, while speech may be restored within a few days, thinking processes may take months or years. In fact, "recovery" does not necessarily imply a full restoration to pre-injury status. It is a more relative term, and more commonly represents a percentage of what abilities a patient once had. Thus, the extent of damage, the location of injury and the recovery process itself are variable in each individual.

Memory Processes

Head injured patients consistently suffer amnesia about events following the injury. Even when a patient is past the PTA described earlier, memory processes are erratic. Sometimes a patient will regain a very specific skill, such as spelling, while experiencing severe deficits across the cognitive domain. As recovery progresses, the patient's recall of earlier learned material is ragged. Generally, quantitative concepts (e.g., measurement, relationships, application of numerical operations) are recalled sooner than number facts or processes in calculation. Single word identification is usually at grade level long before comprehension of reading passages. Math skills may remain intact in the patient with severe aphasia.

Pre-injury Achievement

Added to this variability in injury and recovery rate is the prior academic achievement of each child. Individual learning preferences and differences in achievement have their effect upon what is available for a patient to recall. Existent learning problems will remain; in fact, they more often are exacerbated by the injury.

Treatment Differences

Variability among patients includes differences in the treatment received from the time of emergency care to school readmission. Some patients will be transferred from intensive care units to general hospitals and then discharged to home when their medical status becomes stable. They may, in some cases, experience no difficulty in returning to former activities, including school. Others may be discharged directly to home, where the disruptive and provocative behaviors of agitation, severe amnesia and disorientation—prominent in the early stages of recovery—are played out within the care of the family. During this stage, loss of immediate memory is so severe that returning a patient to school would have no function other than a custodial one. A patient at this stage, for example, might ask repeatedly for accounts of the accident. In one 30 minute segment, a therapist will be asked for the same information several times; and for the duration of the day and evening, even for days thereafter, everyone whom the patient meets will be queried. The patient's need to learn what has happened—and therefore, to remember—is immense, but the vehicle for remembering is insufficient for even this vital information.

Still other patients are discharged from intensive care units to tertiary settings such as rehabilitative units. Their medical, nursing and therapeutic needs take priority over cognitive and educational ones at this time. Admission to this course of treatment presumes that such a resource is available within reasonable distance, at least for weekend visits by families, and that it is accessible (i.e., there must be empty beds). Families must be able to meet a heavy obligation of medical bills with insurance or other resources. For many patients, this type of treatment is not an option.

That patients will not progress without rehabilitation is not argued. Those who can avail themselves of rehabilitation, however, may find quite a difference between its end effects and their readiness for school. For example, the course of recovery and its quality can be influenced by stimulation, intensive therapy, structure and appropriate management during this critical period of rapid change. A patient who receives several treatment therapies a day and is surrounded by a staff who respond to agitated, confused and disorganized behavior in consistent ways may be at less risk of developing maladaptive patterns of physical and psychosocial behavior to carry into school. Families or educators are not expected to have the personal resources, knowledge, or objectivity to care for children at home or in school during this stage of recovery. Even when families can accept intellectually that their children are not responsible for their behavior under these circumstances, they often find a child's behavior painfully embarrassing during the immediate postcoma period; they tend to react in parental, punitive fashion to behaviors such as public masturbation, profanity or aggression. All the years of early training of their youngster for social control appear to have been for nothing. It is much easier for a professional staff member to interpret this lack of control as disinhibition created by injury, and then matter of factly ignore the behavior or instruct the patient that the behavior is inappropriate—confident that as the brain heals, the disinhibition will abate. The same confidence and objectivity are needed by teachers if they face undesirable and inappropriate behaviors when the patient returns to school. The rule of variability dictates that such behavior is not predictable.

Thus school planning, in particular, is made tentative not only by the differences in the rate and progress of recovery of each individual, but by variability in the degree and nature of impairment, in preinjury achievement and intelligence, and in the course of treatment itself.

Structure

There are several needs common to all head injured students that are *not* variable. Head injured students have been subjected to a great deal of structure by virtue of having been patients. Structure is provided in any hospital by the routine administration of care, medication, therapies, meals and visiting hours. In a rehabilitation hospital, the structure is made denser by increased therapies. Many patients have physical therapy and/or occupational therapy three times a day, one half hour each time, and speech therapy twice a day; they also participate in orientation groups, recreational activities and educational tutoring. This tightly scheduled day excludes the need for patients to initiate activities or make decisions. Schedules are adhered to closely and abandoned only for some other activity such as a visit to the X-ray lab or dentist.

Patients with fresh injuries do not organize themselves into constructive occupations. Initiative, motivation, and judgment are absent. Thus, for the immediate weeks after injury and for many weeks beyond, caregivers must provide structure as a vehicle for carrying out daily living activities. This is no less true for school activity. Returning to school with its inherent schedule of classes and activities provides a badly needed routine (structure) within which the patient can function. However, activity must continually be defined more narrowly so that each class in the schedule, each activity in the class, and each assignment in each activity reinforce and develop structure. For example, no returning head injured student is likely to benefit from a period assigned to the library or study hall when independent work is expected. A teacher must organize the class schedule tightly to provide supervision and assistance during every period. Thus students need to be assigned to resource rooms, guidance offices or health rooms instead of study halls.

During instruction, the teacher's written and oral directions need to be specific and task oriented, and clear expectations about the task are required. For example, an elementary teacher can expect low productivity from an assignment asking students to write a composition about the class field trip to the aquarium. Added structure is needed, such as, ''Write about two or three major differences between the seals and the sharks that you observed during your visit to the aquarium. You may focus on their natural habitats, their habitats within the aquarium, their food or habits, characteristics or care. Compositions should be about two pages and at least three paragraphs, and may be handwritten or typed. They are due the day after tomorrow.'' (To the head injured student specifically, the teacher says, ''I would like to see your outline tomorrow.'') Teachers need not fear that they are depriving head injured students by limiting their choices of freedom during this first year of recovery. These students function best when provided with organization, clearly stated expectations, systematic and consistent routine, and limited choices. To appreciate this further, contrast these students with the best students in a class. These superior students can be relied upon to make good judgments about study, work, and play. They can proceed with fewer instructions and details, and can write and work independently much more skillfully than limited students.

To get another sense of structure, imagine trying to determine a building's purpose before it has been completed. Structure might be likened to the stages of preparing this building for use. First come the foundation and walls—a shell (minimal structure, undefined purpose). Then inner walls lend an idea of how the building *might* be used. Equipment further dictates how it *will* be used (e.g., restaurant or office); outlets, appliances, lighting narrow the possibilities still further, and furnishings dictate them further yet. The more that is added to the building, the more clearly defined (or limited) its use. Just as the outer shell of a building tells little about how it will be used upon completion, so the basic schedule of classes tells the head injured student little about how to proceed. But the teacher's continuing definition of structure down to the assignment in front of the student (the furnishings) makes clearer what is required. Head injured students will need the furnishings before they can make a judgment about how to use the room.

Structure, then, is one of the most important invariable needs of head injured students. A discussion of the variety of ways to develop structure and to modify it as students change follows in Chapter 5.

Flexibility

Because of considerable time lost from school, students re-enter without the skills and content covered during their absence. These deficits are compounded by the injury and by memory and processing impairment. Although hospital tutoring is often available, its effectiveness is reduced for the following reasons:

By the time patients have enough memory to begin studying again, it is often almost time to go home.

Tutoring competes with medical and therapeutic attention, and in a medical setting has less priority.

Tutoring may have prepared students somewhat for how difficult learning is about to become, but otherwise it is often
too little, too late to have compensated for the losses.

Thus the school staff must be willing to hold in abeyance
various requirements regarding Carnegie units and credits when
considering placement at the time of the patient's return. Students re-enter school at great disadvantage that requires accom-
modation and time: time to make up what has been missed; time
extended in testing and completion of assignments; time taken
by teachers for repeating directions and giving extra assistance;
time to get from one place to another—in essence, time to recover.
Flexibility is required to strike a balance between accommoda-
tion to requirements and provision for students who are not prepared to join their classes midstream but who should not have
to wait for anything as arbitrary as a new term. Examples of effective staff flexibility are discussed in Chapter 6.

Reduced Demands

In hand with flexibility is the practice of reducing the demands
made upon head injured students. At the secondary level, this
modification in program can take the form of substituting a less
demanding class in the same subject for the one the student was
enrolled in prior to the injury or of substituting totally new subjects for those which require heavy reading or written assignments, abstraction, much memorization or complex language.
The student's reading comprehension and speed are likely to
be well below grade level. For elementary and secondary students alike, extended time limits reduce the quantity of work
to a more achievable task and are integral to achievement during this period of recovery.

Although there are times when students must develop their
decoding skills and reading comprehension skills, there are also
times when information acquisition is the more important goal,
and any way in which a student can acquire information is
acceptable. Thus, parents are encouraged to read material to their
children or to use audiotapes. Students faced with reading novels
for English assignments might use audiotapes to help comprehension. Such tapes are available through state resources for the
blind (also available to students with learning disabilities),

public libraries and through commercial companies such as Books on Tape (1-800-626-3333).

Parents should be cautioned that sometimes their child's listening comprehension is also poor, thereby reducing the value of taped material.

Reducing the demands of testing may dictate that students receive oral tests (perhaps administered by a resource teacher) and extended time limits, or that they be assigned projects to demonstrate the grasp of a skill or concept in lieu of extensive written work. Teachers should construct tests and assignments to measure recognition rather than recall. If given at all, memorization assignments will be more successful if their content is organized for ease in recall. Mnemonics or cues for self-prompting improve a student's memorization and are discussed in more detail in Chapter 4. Although the need for memory in everyday life cannot be ignored, teachers should avoid the use of any rote memory tasks as a measure of whether learning has taken place, because head injured students are at such a disadvantage.

Teachers and parents must modify their expectations that secondary school students be entirely independent and responsible for their work. Head injured students will forget to turn in completed homework, lose their assignments, or fail to write them down in the first place. Their comprehension of spoken language may by very inefficient, requiring that information or directions be repeated or rephrased.

The value of note taking is lost to most head injured students, whose efficiency will be severely reduced by some combination of poor listening comprehension, hemiplegia or weakness in the dominant hand, inability to recognize the most salient information, and distraction. Borrowing the notes of a good student or using notes written on special duplicating papers by good note takers provides students with information that they cannot acquire independently and information that is badly needed by tutors and parents who are trying to help them prepare homework and other assignments.

Supervision

What supervision do head injured students require that is different than other students? In elementary schools where physical space and class size are on a smaller scale, not much more supervision than the ordinary may be required. At the secondary level, the size of physical plant, the number of students in the building and the frequency of social contact among students make supervision much more difficult.

For a weakly oriented student, trips to the lavatory, for example, can be a source of trouble, depending on who else is there. One patient started up conversations with others who were using the facilities and, totally distracted by the conversation, ended up following them back to their classes, only to find himself lost.

The poor judgment and naiveté that are common among head injured students leave them especially susceptible to persuasion and vulnerable to adolescent humor, teasing, and practical jokes. Cafeterias and corridors are mine fields for head injured students, and these areas are the bane of supervision for most staff. Sometimes "buddies" can be prevailed on to help carry books and trays, orient to place, and befriend in the cafeteria. Sometimes, however, befriending a head injured student means jeopardizing one's own social standing, especially if that student's behavior is conspicuous or misunderstood.

An effective use of the guidance staff is to rely on its built-in capability for monitoring and supervising a wide range of student activities. As intermediaries between students and teachers, guidance counselors provide coordination and communication among the various people involved with the student. This service is especially useful in secondary schools. The guidance office is preferable to a study hall and a student assigned there once a day can be given simple tasks to do while a counselor monitors him or her for changes. This also establishes a contact between the student and one key person when general help is needed.

A student's more subtle needs for supervision fall in the realm of teacher planning, whether in organizing daily work or planning for long range assignments. These needs are discussed further in strategies for developing structure.

Intervention

Head injured students are not always conspicuous nor are they always known to teachers, who must become familiar with many students. Early identification of the head injured student's needs has the potential to prevent distress. Without such intervention, the chances of failure, misunderstanding, inappropriate demands and seeming indifference of both staff and student are increased.

Transitions from Hospital to Home

When patients emerge from therapeutic, rehabilitative settings, they have generally recovered memory functions and control of behavior sufficiently to be amenable to participation in school, if only in a limited way. Thus, when this text suggests that immediate return to school be encouraged, it is in reference to patients who have recovered to this extent.

The urgency behind early school return may be questioned, or it might be asked if return to school shouldn't be delayed further until the patient's changing mental status stabilizes still more, for example, particularly since the variability contributes to so much difficulty in school planning.

There are several justifications for this positive attitude toward early return. Patients confront the approaching date of discharge with ambivalence about leaving the hospital. Many have been there long enough to develop attachments to the staff, to become used to the security of a place where their needs are anticipated and met. Eager as a patient may be to leave, the world beyond may seem quite frightening. Eagerness is mixed with dread. Ideally, the patient has spent a few trial weekends at home, and to stay at home for good becomes a goal in itself. Home is viewed as a haven; it can become an escape to one's room, without demands, or outsiders, so comfortable that it may be hard to leave.

If a patient leaves the hospital with the expectation of resuming a "normal" life, then returning to school reinforces a self-perception of normalcy. To be at home is to be in school if the patient is going to fit in with peers. To be at home and not to be in school emphasizes a patient's disability and "differentness," and invites a prolonged self-perception as an invalid. Why contribute to that negative self image? Under these circumstances, it is unlikely that the patient will find returning to school any easier at some future date.

One caveat for parents and teachers: Returning to school is as shaky a step psychologically as it is physically. Children will have lost the comfortable familiarity of friends by being absent for a long time and by wearing the scars and evidence of injury that set them apart. As patients, they have experienced a paradox of "differentness": they are aware of being different from the persons they once were, but they are *not* different from those around them in the hospital.

Finding company in one's difference affords a certain amount of comfort and consolation. Patients root for each other. They can even appreciate that other patients' conditions are worse by comparison. When they venture out into the community during hospital rehabilitation (a planned activity of deconditioning to reduce self-consciousness and fear), they are *together* with others who are different and, therefore, the same. To return to school, however, is to return alone and different—different from the person the student once was and also different from everyone else.

Placement and Programs

Prior to their injury, most head injured children followed a typical developmental course of growth and achievement. In those cases where children have previously encountered problems, parents essentially still considered their children to be average. More to the point, these children were not handicapped at birth. This factor contributes to their uniqueness in that a normal course of development has been interrupted. Parents of suddenly injured children suddenly become parents of handicapped children. As such, they have to acquire very quickly new expectations of what their child can and cannot do. Because the handicap is fresh and parents have had little experience with it, they often inaccurately estimate what is possible.

School staff are equally inexperienced with the handicap of head trauma, largely because of its rarity in the school population. Thus, both parents and educational staff alike may hold unrealistic or uncertain expectations.

As a result, a patient's immediate return to school at the end of hospitalization is often discounted as a possibility. Parents worry about how to transport a wheelchair-bound child to a given destination; even when mobility is not an issue, they wonder whether as working parents they will have time to transport a child obviously unready to ride on an unsupervised school bus. They need to learn a lot about what schools will provide; unaccustomed to planning for a handicapped child, they are unaware of how much is provided.

Educational staff, accustomed to planning for all children, follow very explicit directions for providing services, especially if the student is handicapped. Public Law 94-142 establishes the wherewithal to accommodate head injured students in educational programs. As a mandate for public education for all handicapped students, the law provides the structure by which these students may be assessed for eligibility, determines the extent and nature of the handicap, the ancillary therapeutic services to which children are entitled and a time frame within which they must be provided. Access to these benefits of the law is defined in guidelines by each state in its interpretation of the federal mandate.

PL94-142 lists brain injury among handicapping conditions under learning disability, which in itself is an umbrella for the needs of head injured students. However, the law has to be interpreted generously in order to provide timely services that meet these students' needs. The growing population of brain damaged, traumatically injured surviving children and adolescents who now seek services was not in existence during the years of the development of the law. Their unique needs are not addressed.

For example, the time constraints and qualifying evaluations that are necessary for planning of special education services, designed with intent to protect students from inappropriate placement, sometimes work to the disadvantage of head trauma students.

On one hand, schools need lead time to plan for gathering medical reports, assessments, organization of staff for review and assignment, transportation scheduling and provision of therapies. By law, staff meetings must be held in order to review qualifying data and develop individual educational plans for each aspect of student activity. Prior to these conferences, students must receive achievement and psychologic evaluations.

On the other hand, the nature and course of recovery is unpredictable enough to impede planning in advance. In some children, 2 weeks of recovery will change many of the planning needs. Yet those changes cannot be predicted dependably, and educational plans cannot be developed on the basis of what *might* be needed.

Occasionally, students quickly become ready for discharge, leaving insufficient time to accomplish the required paper work for school readmission especially if special education is needed. Lack of preparation for a student's reentry to school causes valuable loss of time and delays an optimal transition from hospital to home or school.

An important qualifier of Public Law 94-142 for special education is that children must be assigned to the least restrictive school environment needed to accomplish learning. Eligibility for services qualifies students for physical and occupational therapy, speech/language therapy, psychologic counseling, transportation, and special education programming. The range of services begins with minimal intervention such as the consultation of an occupational therapist with the classroom teacher about the needs of a given student; it extends to full-time placement within a residential school. Philosophically, the law reflects the need and right of handicapped children to learn in the most normal setting possible. The classroom must be one in which the handicap is minimized and strengths are maximized. A handicap is in itself not a sufficient reason to exclude children from the normal course of life. Thus, "mainstreaming" as a concept requires vigilance against setting apart handicapped students from others or restricting their opportunities to associate with nonhandicapped students. To the extent possible, students are placed in standard classrooms for as much instruction as can be utilized there, and are assigned to resource classrooms for only those periods in which remedial instruction is needed.

It may be that a student's deficits are severe enough to warrant a full-time placement in a self-contained classroom, or even in a special wing or unit apart from the main stream. If so, the law provides such; if not, the law safeguards against undue isolation and limitation of movement within regular schools.

Comparison with Other Handicapping Conditions

Designated handicapping conditions often do not accurately describe head trauma students. Thus, instructional environments, although noncategorical in some school systems (that is, classes are not arranged by disability), are often tailored to respond to particular handicaps, and therefore are not necessarily appropriate. For example, the labels "learning disability" and "multi-handicapped" are expedient but not accurately descriptive of closed head injured students. Certainly, cognitive deficits are present but these are uneven in the extent of damage and in the rate of recovery. More importantly, these deficits are preceded by achievement that is unlike that of children who are developmentally delayed. There are visual-perceptual deficits and hemianopsia that contribute to vision-related problems in learning, but for which placement in a vision-impaired program would be inappropriate. Although reading comprehension may be well below age and grade level at the time of reentry into school, head injured students may recover previous reading skills. Techniques for teaching a nonreader are not necessarily applicable to teaching a reader how to recover prior reading skills. Classes for students with learning disabilities provide smaller teacher-pupil ratios and more supervision and structure, but they may lack the cognitive intervention head injured students need.

The variability present in cognitive recovery is also present in motor recovery. Some students return to school in wheelchairs; others have no visible impairment. The extent of cognitive impairment and the long range need for therapies are other factors that impinge on variability and complicate placement decisions. These are some of the problems that emerge:

- Students who require extensive therapies are most often accommodated in central locations where full-time therapists and specialized equipment provide therapies two to three times a week.
- Many of the non–head injured students who require this much therapy require lifelong therapies and services because they are severely involved motorically and often experience not only motor impairment but also speech, language, and cognitive impairment.
- Head injured students may have similar motor disability but they require intensive physical and occupational therapy for a short period of time (the average is a few months).

• Although this setting may be appropriate from a logistical point of view, it is inappropriate from a social and educational point of view because the non–head injured children are not peers.

Thus, the demand for short range, intensive therapy is not easily accommodated by a system whose primary purpose is education. For secondary students who require less but regular treatment, there are few resources of therapy within the schools. For elementary students, there is more likely to be limited therapy available. Other agencies (e.g., the Health Department or Visiting Nurse Association) are called upon to help older students.

Ironically, children who are mildly damaged and are in wheelchairs temporarily or not at all, and who do not fit multi-handicapped, restrictive settings, actually face a more complicated placement decision. Further, students are occasionally penalized at the time of return to school if they must attend a different school in order to gain wheelchair access, thereby losing friends and familiar teachers.

Comparison with Psychiatric Patients

Children who receive psychiatric services under PL94-142 are labeled emotionally disturbed or emotionally handicapped. These students are likely to have had a history of behavioral, emotional or learning difficulty subsequent to their injury. The socially inappropriate, out-of-control behaviors of some head injured students certainly resemble those of certain emotionally disturbed students. And indeed, some head injury does result in long term psychiatric disturbance. For the most part, however, poor judgment and loss of control are temporary effects of head injury.

Placement

Although many head injured students qualify for special education services as handicapped students, many are served well by mainstreaming and a small percentage require no special education. Most do need some kind of intervention, if only to have someone monitor, direct and supervise activity. Ideally, the strengths of both special education and mainstreaming should be utilized.

Given the special education law, the variety of pupil needs and the variety of resources in any one school system, there is no one model placement or program. Each student's placement has to be considered individually.

The following options and their frequency (listed in Table 4-1) demonstrate the variety of placement decisions made for the Kennedy Institute population of head injured students from 1981 to 1984.

Home Instruction

In Maryland, a minimum of 4 weeks of need must be assured because of the administrative cost and effort of arranging for home tutors. A maximum number of 6 hours a week can be received in home instruction. Students are not given home instruction in addition to school instruction. Home teaching is not to be confused with enrichment teaching, but utilized as a substitute to school instruction rather than a supplement.

Combination of Home and School

This is not a contradiction of the above statement. When home instruction is used with school visits, the school visits are for socialization only. One student, for example, visited the school at lunch time each day and included a brief homeroom activity that followed lunch. Occupational therapy was given before the return home to a tutor later in the afternoon. Somewhere in that schedule the student took a nap. Newly discharged patients often fatigue easily and need rest interspersed during the day, even when they are beyond the typical age for napping.

Reduced School Program

In line with the need for rest is the need for low doses of activities that require concentration. The patient's gradual return to school is in keeping with the gradual return of function. It may be that a student will only participate a few hours for a very short time (e.g., as little as 2 weeks) before resuming a day-long schedule. Then the reduced program will have to take place

Table 4–1.   Frequency of Educational Options Available Upon Discharge

Option	% of Study Population	Number of Students
Home instruction		
Min. 4 weeks, max. 6 hrs/wk (in Maryland)	10	7
Combination home/school		
Informal school visits and home teaching	5	4
Reduced school program		
One/two periods a day, with resource teacher	3	2
Modified school program		
Substitution of less demanding classes; private tutor; assistance from guidance staff	8	6
Special education programs		
Mainstream with resource help; academic level maintained	15	11
Self-contained special ed classrooms	4	3
Special schools or wings	10	7
Residential schools	0	0
No return to school		
6 were high school graduates; 5 were comatose	20	14
No services, return to same class	15	11
No services, repeat of grade	3	2
Unknown	5	4
Total	98	71

within the confines of the school day. The reduced day may include time with a resource teacher or time in a relatively undemanding class or a combination of both. How does one decide on these options? For starters, the student's cognitive return will govern most decisions. The extent of his or her motor handicap will play a part. Mundane issues of whether a desired class fits within the schedule or is located nearby or whether stairs have to be negotiated can enter into the decision.

Modified School Program

A modified program differs from a reduced one in that students will be in school for the entire day as opposed to a reduced day. Then less demanding classes are substituted and resources other than the teaching staff are called upon. There have been a number of creative options worked out for students in this regard.

In one instance, the student's family paid for a private tutor to work with their son during the school day. A returning senior who had not met the junior year requirement for a paper in English worked privately with the tutor to fill this requirement while keeping up with senior year English. Another was tutored the first half of the year in Algebra I in order to be ready to take the second half with the class. This was a volunteer effort of the teacher, who used her free period and the student's resource period to accomplish this. This is a good example of the extent to which people will exert themselves to help these students, particularly when the student has been a good student and an achiever.

In addition to tutors, school or private, the guidance staff is another resource for helping develop a modified day and for participating in supervision during some part of the day.

Special Education Programs

In keeping with the mandate to provide education in the least restrictive environment, it is preferable to place students in their home schools and supply help from a resource teacher for those areas of difficulty that remain. Some students can maintain academic levels with this amount of support. Others have deficits that are pervasive enough to warrant being in a self-contained classroom for all subjects. Occasionally students in these classrooms are able to join a regular classroom for lunch, gym or art. Students with more complicated learning problems are assisted by special education teachers in special wings or schools. This physical isolation from the standard classroom is an acknowledgment that the student's problems of learning and behavior are too severe to be managed in a regular class for even a short time. Except for a residential school, this is the most restrictive setting.

No Services; Return to Same Class

It is important to remember that not all head injured students have severe deficits. Some do return to school without further intervention. Of this group, some needed services but were not given them. This is in part attributable to the demands of the law. A verifiable handicap must be identified. The deficits must be severe enough to warrant special education. In addition, even though a student's difficulty can be predicted, it is not always possible to provide what is needed or to judge what will prevent the difficulty. For example, one student in this population was required to return to the ninth grade because he had missed a half year of school. Summer school had not been an option because of the timing of his hospital discharge. He was an intelligent but uneven-achieving student. In the school's judgment it was best that he review and learn by repeating the ninth grade but it was the student's opinion that that was the last place he wanted to be. He hated school, most of his teachers, and spoke disparagingly of his peers. The problems were very predictable at that time, but the solutions escaped those planning for his return. His first few months back at school erupted into a no-win situation until the escalating behavior fit the criteria for special education, and he was placed in a special school for students with psychiatric problems.

Chapter 5

Instructional Preparation

PREPARATION

By now, teachers and parents should have a good sense of the *person* who is recovering from brain injury and some idea of the problems that person will present as a student.

How do teachers prepare mentally for the demands that head injured students will make upon them? For starters:

- Teachers must accept the fact of a child's placement in their classrooms.

Often teachers have little say about who is assigned to their classes, but strong feelings about the task of managing any very difficult child need to be acknowledged, at least mentally. The attitude that any student should be someone else's responsibility sabotages most constructive approaches to teaching. The authors' experience has been that many teachers can identify with the unfortunate circumstances of severe injury and give their best. But when unwillingness and resentment prevail, perhaps the ultimate prod is to ask, "What kind of help would I want *my* child to have?"

- The reality is that not all students are likable and some head injured students are less likable than others.

Sometimes teachers need to step back a little from the intensity of the situation to regain perspective. That is also a time they need exceptional support from the administration and other staff members. Some of that support takes the form of recognition from the administration, release time for courses and workshops, consultation with others who can assist, and certainly acknowledgment in the form of merit pay.

* Not all head injured students present enormous problems but a few are very trying and require patience, ingenuity, and perseverance nearly beyond the call of duty.

Head injured students commonly recover within 6 months to a year many skills which had become automatic prior to their injury. Skills such as decoding, encoding, short passage comprehension, and elementary quantitative processes generally return.

* The problem of memory impairment is not so much the retrieval of previously learned skills but gaining short term memory for new learning. Much of the old learning will reemerge with review. The importance of this should not be overlooked.

REVIEW VERSUS NEW LEARNING

Educators are accustomed to conceptualizing learning as a hierarchical process in which one thing builds on another and skills at a basic level are taught (and learned) before going on to more advanced skills and concepts. This concept of learning is less applicable to head injured students whose short term memory loss may impede learning of rote material but whose long term memory may enable conceptual recall. For example, one student conceptualized set theory and division in math, but failed to recall number facts during daily drills. Another could appreciate the values of food groups but could not list all the foods that contained a specific vitamin.

* Overlearning, or repeated study and drill to increase the length of time something will be remembered, does not have the same value in the review of previously learned information as it does during initial learning.

If a student demonstrates adequate conceptualization of previously learned material during a given exercise in which mastery is the goal, no further drill is necessary.

- Once a head injured student demonstrates that he or she can retrieve previously learned material, teachers can rely on this as evidence that learning has taken place.

New learning is quite another matter. Not all injured students exhibit all deficits and those they do form unique clusters of compounded deficits that impinge on each other. For example, memory is a mix of short term, long term, semantic, episodic and immediate memories that interact with attention, awareness, perception, thinking and understanding of rote materials, discourse, spoken and written language comprehension, encoding and decoding functions, mathematics, and so on. Combined with the many facets of memory are other aspects of cognition: judgment, impulsivity, associativeness, concreteness, and perseveration. Thus any one child has some combination of capabilities and deficits that interact with one another to which teachers must respond (always observing, not predicting, vigilant for evidence of change).

In addition to mental preparation for these unusual students, what prior education and experience prepare teachers for teaching memory-impaired students?

LEARNING THEORY

One of the best sources of review appears to be the body of research and theory about how individuals learn (or don't learn!). Endemic to head-injured students is some degree of cognitive impairment. Because they are inefficient learners of new information, they must lean upon many external strategies for learning, retention and recall.

An information processing model offers a guide to the task the learner faces: getting information in, retaining it, and retrieving it when it is needed. Perception and selective attention, or focus, are active initially. In addition, the way material is organized has an effect on how well a person remembers and recalls it.

Transference research has also shown that the activity that precedes and follows study may facilitate or interfere with what is learned and whether it is generalized. Other principles such as the *serial position effect*, the *role of reinforcement*, and a large body of observations and studies provide direction for efficient learning. If a student prepares for an exam by reading lengthy material, his or her memory for that material will be greater if the activity that directly follows is in contrast. An example would be walking or jogging after studying history rather than reading in a similar subject. Otherwise the second reading tends to blur the concepts studied in the first (retroactive inhibition). Some kinds of learning reinforce prior learning (retroactive facilitation). For example, the use of new vocabulary words in context reinforces the study of vocabulary definitions.

Studies in serial position effect show that subjects given a list of items to remember recall first those at the beginning and the end, while the ones in the middle are usually forgotten. This principle underscores the importance of primacy (first in the list) and recency (the last or most recent item). Thus teachers must continually rearrange the order in which things are grouped during learning so that items fall in a different sequence.

Organization

Students can benefit further from instruction when material is organized for efficient storage and retrieval in the form of a summary or when it is organized simultaneously with an outline as a structure for note taking. It is not enough that a lesson has been well organized for teacher presentation. The organization needs to be made obvious to students, so that the process becomes a model for their own adoption.

Information presented in advance of a lesson as brief cues to what will follow often helps gain students' attention and alerts them to the most important information that the teacher is going to present. Conceived as "advanced organizers" by Ausubel (1960), the use of such clues is prevalent in instructional technology such as computer-assisted instruction, but is also commonly used when teachers being a lesson with, "Today we are going to discuss winter holidays."

Motivational study or presenting students with central clues around which to categorize or sort information in advance of study teaches them to relate that instruction to the advance organizers while identifying key concepts. Recall of organized information is made easier by the association of ideas with each other. Recall of one concept provokes memory of a related concept, especially if those concepts are learned in relation to each other.

The use of mnemonic strategy is valuable for memorizing unrelated concepts or information. The most common mnemonic devices are those of memorized verses (e.g., "30 days hath September" or the use of the rhyme "one, bun, two, shoe, three, tree"). An alternate method is the use of a very familiar building (e.g., a person's house) in which items are graphically stored in various rooms. A mental walk through the rooms provides recall of the items "placed" in each. There are some clarifications to the method, which are noted by Bower (1970). Students should be taught to use the same "house" or scene each time they memorize. The house or "cues" should be available to the student at the time the list of items is being committed to memory. Head injured students may benefit from being presented with external pictures to use for recall. The external cues may be devised by the person who is helping the student although, when possible, encouraging the student to generate personal images is preferred. These external cues may need to be presented at the time of recall as well as at the time of memorization.

One aside here: Students cannot be expected to develop a system by themselves, and the establishment of a system of cues takes the time and skill of some other person, whether parent, teacher, guidance counselor or resource staff. Once a system has been established, a student should use the same device, and by doing so gradually diminish the need for supervision during study.

A particular student comes to mind to illustrate how this might be used. An eighth grader returned to school assigned to a cooking class, a choice believed to be less stressful than a subject with heavy reading and complex concepts. She faced an early challenge of learning all the foods that contain vitamin C—a rote memory task she failed and for which she could not be held responsible, given her short term memory deficits. Had she used a mnemonic device and been allowed external cues for recall, her performance might have improved. What follows is an example of a step-by-step plan for developing a mnemonic device which could have been used with this student:

Begin a memory imprint of a series of loci or places, such as the student's home, the school, or any very familiar building that has a number of rooms with a variety of detail: windows, doors, and so forth. A park or setting other than a building can be used as long as it is well known and has enough variety to distinguish different loci.

After helping the student to decide on the building, or loci, the resource person writes down a brief description of each room as dictated by the student. Then, using a seed catalog, both gather pictures of the actual fruits and vegetables to be memorized. The student will then need help in placing each fruit or vegetable in a room, creating a ludicrous or unusual image (e.g., a bunch of broccoli in the door knocker, carrots arranged as a bouquet or a TV antenna). After placing each thing to be learned throughout the loci, the student reviews the placements, always moving through the rooms or loci in the same order. This way, the student can determine which room was omitted, for which room an item could not be recalled, or which items could be recalled in isolation. If the student has difficulty remembering the order of the rooms or loci, a cue card with this order should be available. The student may need this same external cue card during an exam. If the name of the room in itself is not enough of a cue, then the object or place in the room could serve as a prompt (e.g., the door knocker, a vase on the mantel, and so on).

Essentially what such a system accomplishes is the provision of "pigeon holes" or files and a retrieval scheme which gives the student some structures for where and how to begin recall, how to move from one item to the next, how to determine when an item has been overlooked, and when the list has been completed.

This system, once developed, should be retained by the student for future memory tasks. Then the cues (or loci) would be available at the time any new list of items was studied. A series on 3 x 5 cards to use as future reference would preserve the system for further use. Using this basic device, a student can develop more sophisticated uses such as chronological events in history, sequential events in a lab procedure, or series of points for an essay. (To that end, all students could benefit from being taught how to develop their personal schemata for retrieval of information.)

Other Learning

What does new learning require of a student besides memory? Study is also required; before that, planning, and before that, understanding the assignment and attention to the task. Before students can remember anything they have to get it into short term memory: first, by way of attention and focus, then by search or scanning techniques, finally by organizing material for retention and eventual retrieval. Underlying all of these skills is the awareness or *knowledge* that a person knows something or does not. Coined "secondary ignorance" by Sieber (1968) or conceptualized as metacognition by Flavell (1970) and Brown (1975), the condition of not knowing is pervasive among the head injured: not knowing they do not understand, not knowing the limits of their memories, not knowing how to ascertain the state of their ignorance. If head injured students could walk up to their teachers and say, "Look, I've had a brain injury and I won't be able to memorize that list of things," transitions might be smoother. But they're not likely to do this for a number of reasons: embarrassment, weak self-esteem, not wanting to call attention to their deficits and weaknesses, fear of ridicule or punishment. However many reasons might explain this inability, the most probable is that *reduced metacognition is paramount*. The ability of learners to monitor their own progress, weaknesses, and achievement is integral to planning for learning.

Cognitive strategies (or planning for learning) are thought by Gagne (1979) to be developed by an internal control process in which learners select and modify what they attend to, what they will remember and how they will do so, gradually developing management of their own thinking. For head injured students particularly, control is a major issue. For some, loss of control is manifested in poor gross or fine motor activity. More overtly, they lose control over their lives and activity by the fact of the injury itself. Often control over eating, social behavior, and thinking is diminished. Thus, the development or reestablishment of internal control is an ambitious task for head injured students and one that is made more difficult by the injury.

Attention to this will not be wasted on others in the class, however, for many students need assistance with learning to learn. Although students have been learning how to learn while they have been learning other things, some have learned more efficiently than others. All but the best students require continuing help in developing internal cognitive strategies by first using external strategies which eventually become internalized and later can be applied when needed.

Adaptations

A common residual motor deficit is weakness on one side of the body (hemiparesis). If this weakness happens to be on the dominant side, then writing skills will be considerably altered, sometimes to the extent of needing to change hands for writing. Frequently writing speed is slow and the legibility poor. Technology and ingenuity have produced many sophisticated mechanical and electronic adaptive devices that provide mobility, self-care and independence.

If these are not available, providing a note taker or scribe is one way to assist students with information that has to be written while in class. Special self-copying papers will facilitate the process. Of course, there are always tape recorders, but the noise level in the classroom often interferes with clear recording. Students have to listen to long segments of the tape to find particular items, and tape recorders are awkward to carry, especially if a person has only one good side at best.

"Buddies" help students find their way around a building and lend physical support such as carrying books or lunches. A buddy system also provides badly needed social support and interaction.

Allowance needs to be made for head injured students' reduced speed in navigating corridors during class changes. Generally, an advance dismissal of a few minutes is sufficient.

BEHAVIOR AND PSYCHOLOGIC MANAGEMENT

Behavior management techniques have proven to be useful in helping head injured students develop self-control. To a large extent, loss of self control is a function of the injury. Hyperphagia, disinhibition, perseveration, and silliness are all evidence of the loss of control. The authors maintain that structure is needed for head injured students, and behavior techniques are one way to provide that structure. For example, one 15 year old boy interrupted inappropriately, spoke out in class and was generally disruptive. A token system was devised that in itself was the structure he needed to stay in control. When the desired behavior was made specific and the consequences tied to something he wanted (reinforcing), he managed to check himself and comply with the request for better classroom behavior. Another boy, 11 years old and wheelchair-bound, was extremely manipulative in trying to avoid physical therapy. Ultimately the entire team had to be informed of the behavior and then united in consistent responses to that behavior. When several teachers have contact with a student, they must communicate frequently so that they can agree upon procedures and respond consistently. The behavior management principles remain the same:

- Ignore unwanted behavior; reinforce desired behavior; guard against reinforcing the very behavior that is unwanted.

Behavior is reinforced simply by giving it attention; avoid doing so when possible. Intervention is most effective when rules are made clear, unwanted behavior is ignored and praise is combined with feedback about performance. If a teacher's praise is not rewarding, then something else must be found as a reinforcer. Other management systems can be tried, such as self-management (student's self-assessment and recording of behavior), peer-mediated feedback (reduction of disapproval statements by the teacher and private feedback to the target student, as well as peer feedback), and time-out procedures (removal from an activity). For more precise description of these techniques, see Strain and Kerr (1981).

A structured environment is also maintained by small teacher-pupil ratios. For some head injured students, large groups of people contribute to confusion and distraction. A small class in itself is not necessarily appropriate; close supervision is required and all activity must be goal directed. There cannot be large blocks of ''free'' time.

For students with severe psychologic and behavior problems, consulting psychologists and psychiatrists can be valuable. Guidance counselors are key people as facilitators of communication among the family, teachers and therapists of the student.

All of the staff and family require assistance in paving the way each day, by identification of frustration levels, provision of fail-safe activity and readily available support.

Chapter **6**

Applications

The educational staff is unlikely to be helped much by the results of intelligence or achievement tests given to head injured students during the earliest period of recovery. Performance at that time is so variable and the interaction of the deficits so unpredictable that interpretation of what the scores mean is rendered very tentatively. Yet these scores are presented at planning conferences; although they reflect damage, they form a poor basis on which to plan. A different kind of measure is needed so educators can perceive more clearly the behavior and needs of head injured students. A continuum of deficits and an accompanying continuum of responses to the deficits is found in Table 6–1, to be used to determine a student's qualitative performance within a range of behaviors. These behaviors should be conceptualized along a continuum of recovery and growth on which a student can be located. Each stage is incremental and implies improvement over previous stages, although, as in any stage theory, individuals occasionally exhibit behaviors that overlap.

First, some cautions:

- These are the most common behaviors witnessed in the early stages of recovery of children and adolescents.
- They may be quite temporary, but in the meantime they are too urgent to be ignored.

Table 6–1. Continuum of Deficits

JUDGMENT		
Careless about safety; impulsive	Very easily persuaded by others; interacts inappropriately	Drives too soon; engages in physical activity too soon; uses alcohol and drugs

MOTIVATION		
Very dependent on others to plan, to engage in activity; exhibits truancy or high absenteeism	Less dependent but less compliant for expected behaviors (e.g., attending class, completing work)	Lacking initiative

SELF-CONTROL		
Overtly disinhibited, (e.g., incidents of masturbation, stealing food, profanity, aggressive behavior, inappropriate affection); emotionally labile	Moderately disinhibited; jokes inappropriately; crude; socially familiar; overreactive, outspoken, talkative; loses temper	Rude; silly; appears immature for age group; is immature; verbally aggressive; sometimes escalates to fighting

SELF-MONITORING		
Dresses carelessly; shows poor hygiene	Perseverative: has tics, mannerisms, repeats same phrases, gets "stuck"	Reads social and non-verbal cues or others' responses poorly; is preoccupied with minor problems

MOOD AND SELF-ESTEEM		
Has low affect; emotionally labile; little awareness of self	Depressed (sad/fatigued); reduced energy; aware of handicap; shows perplexibility; avoids public places; irritable	Sometimes suicidal; sometimes manic; willing to venture out; exhibits self-doubt; hesitant

COMPLIANCE		
Demonstrates outright refusal; responds with verbal outbursts or physical aggression to requests or demands; runs away; is truant	Argumentative; covers up noncompliance; pretends innocence, confusion; is truant from some classes	Manipulative; noncompliant in effect but more subtle: no overt refusals but requests are not met

Table 6–1 (continued).

THINKING	
Easily distracted; loses train of thought; focuses poorly; looks "blank"; thinks very concretely, literally; has poor attention	Shows poor abstraction, especially in language (e.g., proverbs), inference, drawing conclusions; unable to consolidate
READING: SPEED, COMPREHENSION	
Reads very slowly with comprehension well below grade level	Reads at moderate speed; identifies single words at grade level, but comprehends at least two grades below
	May comprehend close to grade level but speed is slow enough to penalize
MATH: FACTS AND APPLICATION	
Has poor memory for facts and processes; shows poor application and understanding of language in word problems; very confused	Exhibits fair application but poor memory for facts; may recall facts but forgets processes; has partial recall
	Displays poor abstract reasoning in word problems; evidences distaste and frustration with processes such as long division with three divisors.
WRITING: SPEED, LEGIBILITY	
Does not write at all; cannot use writing efficiently; may be able to learn to type	Writes too slowly for preparation of work; has poor fine-motor dexterity; may have apraxia
	Demonstrates moderate speed but poor legibility
AUDITORY PROCESSING	
Processes spoken language very inadequately; comprehends well below grade and age level; unable to follow oral directions, even in one to one communication	Improved one to one communication; markedly deficient in oral language comprehension
	Easily overloaded by amounts of oral information usually presented during classroom instruction
VISUAL AND PERCEPTUAL ORGANIZATION	
Suffers from field cuts, blurred vision, and poor depth perception	Lacks spatial organization (e.g., has difficulty lining up figures, columns in math, and so on)
	Plans use of space poorly, (e.g., on paper)

- Not all behaviors will apply across the board.
- Not every student begins at the lowest point and improves; some enter midway.

The continuum provides three general grades of behavior and an accompanying continuum of responses. The major purpose is to provide a profile of needs as a guide for instruction and management. One reminder: although thinking cannot be totally isolated from its components of attention, memory, auditory perception, judgment, and so on, there is some utility in distinguishing thinking processes, for example, from those that are largely memory processes for the purpose of measurement. The same is true of social behavior as apart from cognitive behavior. Users of the continuum need to keep in mind that there is much overlap, while using the most overt behaviors as a guide to understanding the more subtle deficits.

The rationale for using a deficit model is based on the freshness of injury and the temporary and elusive status of many of the deficits. Once a student's recovery extends beyond the deficits in this continuum, the support group should turn to an affirmative model for identification of strengths.

Once a student's strengths are sought, more quantitative measures can be employed to assess achievement and cognitive recovery. Standardized measures are useful in assessing individual changes as opposed to comparing students with norms. Because there will be so much variability within one individual, many facets of an achievement should be observed: single word identification (as opposed to vocabulary); word attack skills; short passage reading; long paragraph reading (memory deficits enter here); comprehension as measured when the student must recall information without reference to the text, and comprehension when the text is available for review. Quantitative skills will need to be evaluated with the same penchant for detection: Are failures in written calculation a function of inadequate memory for number facts or failure to recall processes? Or is the difficulty related to the student's inability to write, since writing and thinking are so interactive? Failure to solve word problems may be failure to comprehend the language in the problem rather than failure to reason. If, for example, a child doesn't correctly carry out a three step calculation presented orally, does that mean the child can't add 4 and 6 and divide by 2, then subtract 3? Or does it mean rather that memory for the components of the direction is poor? Writing speed, when simply copying, will need to be assessed. Moreover, ability to copy from a near point may differ from the ability to copy from a distance.

In what ways can standard test results be helpful to the classroom teacher?

- First, compare results of a current assessment with the pre-injury achievement of the student found in periodic, standard group tests such as the Iowa battery. Note how long after the injury and coma/PTA the current tests were administered. This information should be stated in the beginning of the report. If these tests were administered within the first 6 months of injury, there is likely to be much change.
- Contrast the pre-injury test scores with performance as measured in grades and report card information. Is there a history of failure, difficulty in a certain area, erratic performance, or underachievement?
- Note areas of strength and weakness in the current assessment and contrast with pre-injury assessment. Consider which areas require visual and perceptual skills, which are memory-based skills, which are conceptual, and so forth. Consult the school psychologist for help in interpretation of the subtest scores. Consult other specialists such as language therapists who can shed light on the results of their tests as they apply to the student's overall academic functioning.
- Combine anecdotal information about a student's attitude, work habits, apparent motivation and self-esteem with the record of school attendance. Look for patterns of achievement and failure.

Keep in mind that head injured students are not likely to be better than they were prior to injury. Sometimes the expectation exists that, with a new opportunity to relearn, students will achieve in areas previously proven weak. This does not happen. Rather, previously weak areas tend to be weaker. In 46 percent of the Kennedy Institute population, patients had experienced problems in learning prior to the injury as measured by poor grades, underachievement, repeat of grade, resource instruction, poor attendance, truancy and dropping out of school.

As teachers gather the above information together, they can then proceed to target areas for remediation and review. It is helpful to remember that some skills are automatic (single word identification, letter identification for older students, for example) and will return first. Strengths should be used to approach weaknesses but the history of problem areas cannot be overlooked. To illustrate: one 16 year old girl in the Kennedy Institute population had been in an LD class for several years and had read at only third grade level prior to her injury. Third grade skills for this student represented a return to prior levels of cognitive functioning, whereas for a high achiever this would serve as evidence of severe deficit. Anecdotal reports of a student's style give a clue to some behaviors that will emerge again upon return to school. Teachers can be assured that these behaviors will be more prominent. The high achiever or hard-working student will continue to labor, while the indifferent student will find school no more enticing than it was before the injury. Teachers should spare themselves anguish over the problems that existed before these students' injuries and put their efforts into the strengths.

For purposes of viewing the interaction of various components of cognitive and behavioral processes in the continuum, each will be discussed in more detail. The utility of the continuum should be more obvious after this discussion.

Judgment

Consider some of the major components of judgment: intelligence, critical thinking, self-control. In the early stages of recovery, patients' judgment is often very poor. This is shown by indifference to safety, as when patients are careless on the stairs, or when they attempt to walk without crutches before they're ready. Occasionally adolescent patients return to the unit after a weekend pass and report that they have driven the family car or lifted weights or engaged in some other inappropriate activity. Ordinarily, good judgment would be expected to override a lack of self-control if such existed in individuals. But more commonly the interaction between poor judgment and disinhibition contributes to fighting, impulsive behavior, and unwise disregard for rules, safety or health. (Sometimes the poor judgment rests in the family as well, as when they offer or permit alcohol, even though parents are advised to prohibit the use of alcohol and other drugs during the recovery period.) Generally, by the time patients move to the next stage, they take more care in ambulation, particularly if they have continuing weakness in the limbs. Poor judgment is now more obvious in inappropriate social behavior. The ready acceptance of others' ideas without critical assessment ("Let's steal a car") may persist through the last stage of this continuum for some individuals. Many who can resist outlandish proposals by others are still susceptible to more "reasonable" persuasion. For example, one college freshman, without considering the consequences, left school 2 days before final exams to go home with a friend who lived several hundred miles away. Others may not be vulnerable to this level of persuasion but may exert poor judgment about using alcohol and drugs. Some return to the social activity of partying and engage in the same behavior that put them into the hospital in the first place (i.e., drinking and driving or riding with drinking drivers). Of course lack of judgment is not uncommon among the non–head injured. It does show, however, that experience doesn't always improve judgment.

How will the classroom teacher be helped by knowing an individual's level of judgment? If a student is still indifferent to personal safety, then supervision and assignment to restricted areas will be required. Classes that use tools or chemicals will have to be avoided and physical education will have to be planned more carefully. At the secondary level, freedom to move around the school unsupervised will have to be weighed. Absences from a class will have to be verified against daily absence from school. Generally, unsupervised visits to the library or some other part of the school should be discouraged.

Self-Control

It has been stated that loss of self-control (disinhibition) is a direct result of head trauma. The most extreme forms are present as patients emerge from coma. Disinhibited patients swear a *lot*; they masturbate publicly; they are often very agitated and aggressive. However, it is unlikely that students will arrive at school in this shape. By that time, profanity will be reduced to its usual frequency and the other behaviors will be self-monitored for appropriateness. One behavior that may remain is overeating as the result of an insatiable appetite. Hyperphagia is responsible for food stealing and obesity. As the patient regains self-control, the hyperphagia becomes more manageable. One patient's family had to put locks on the cupboards and refrigerator as safeguards against food stealing in the middle of the night. This patient's teachers reported that 3 years after the accident he was still first at the table whenever there was a social function. However, moving from a locked cupboard to being first in line, small an increment as it is, is progress to the second level of self-control.

Other aspects of the middle level of control show up in inappropriate joking and crudeness among the adolescent population. An undisguised interest in sex and body function spurts out of control in the most inappropriate places—the principal's office or during the middle of class instruction, much to the chagrin of teachers who are trying to maintain classroom control.

Not all students will follow this pattern. Other forms of lack of control show up in social interactions on the street. For example, one 17 year old patient spoke to everyone in the elevator indiscriminately and approached people on the street by introducing himself. Another 16 year old girl hugged people inappropriately. One 5 year old boy kissed the hand of everyone with whom he came in contact. Sometimes poor control over temper is the form this behavior takes.

As control resumes, a student's behavior improves but vestiges of inordinate silliness or immaturity might remain. Coupled with possible poor judgment, these behaviors make students especially vulnerable to scuffles, verbal or physical. Such behavior puts a lot of demand on a teacher. If these students are placed in small special education classes, the interaction with other students who may have similar difficulties is compounded. Administrators have to consider the makeup of the class and the built-in structure when considering how best to provide for these students. Teachers will need to provide much structure to keep the classroom an instructional environment and will need to employ a behavior management program consistently.

Compliance

It is timely to discuss the issue of compliance when discussing behaviors that directly impinge on classroom management. At the lowest level of compliance there is none, but be assured that students who are this noncompliant are more likely to be assigned to very restrictive settings (e.g., residential schools). Because the law protects children against inappropriate placement, it is possible that a very noncompliant student will be given a chance in a regular school program first. Schools do not tolerate physically aggressive, noncompliant students for very long. Either the student improves quickly or is suspended from school. Thus the second level of compliance deserves explanation, since it is from this state that many classroom problems evolve.

Students sometimes cover up their noncompliance by pretending innocence or confusion. They are often argumentative in the classroom, even while being reasonably courteous (and exasperating). They can take up a lot of a teacher's attention doing this, and indeed, the behavior may have some elements of regaining control.

At the third stage of this behavior, much more manipulation is observable and represents a more subtle form of noncompliance, for which teachers can be grateful because it represents progress. These gradations of behavior are difficult to interpret because it is not always clear that these students understand what is expected or that they remember accurately. One student was judged to be indifferent to a teacher's rule that he return to the classroom immediately after using the bathroom. He was not really being belligerent but was distracted by whomever he met there. Another student pretended to be lost whenever he was discovered in a part of the school where his friends were. Enough discoveries of that sort provide evidence of intent rather than confusion but they are not always so consistent. Teachers are not alone in their distaste for being manipulated. Given that manipulation is a common behavior, protection against ambiguous situations may be provided by teachers' maintaining frequent contact among themselves.

Motivation

Ultimately, the level of motivation may be influenced by the physical location of damage as well as by other factors. Patients with frontal lobe injury often experience long term inability to carry out the executive functions required in autonomous behavior. Kirby (1984) notes that the neuropsychological basis of planning in the frontal lobes has been well recognized for about a century and that continuing research studies delineate further the major function of the frontal lobes to be the selection and regulation of cognitive planning. In the early stages of recovery, motivation is moot. Patients are highly dependent upon the nursing staff and become accustomed to having all choices made for them. This dependence may still exist for students who return to school with disability and the experience of a prolonged hospital stay. Moreover, impairment of memory and thinking contributes to much perplexity and competes unfavorably with achievement. It is small wonder that motivation is poor. Changes in physical dependence may improve motivation, but mental work is still exhausting and the adjustment to school is difficult. For some patients, every act must be directed long after they have re-mastered the skills of dressing, feeding, and self-care. Indeed, the criterion for successful self-care is the ability to engage in that activity without direction. Some patients know how to dress and feed themselves but do not do so until directed and some need frequent direction. Seriously impaired students may level off at this state. They may express no initiative, or having demonstrated a wish to accomplish something, may lack the initiative to carry it out.

Self-Monitoring

Patients must reach minimum levels of awareness to monitor their appearance, but sometimes this self-monitoring is also affected by self-control and judgment. One of the most troublesome students at the Kennedy Institute failed to pay attention to dress. Obesity from hyperphagia contributed to his untidiness, as did poor memory, which contributed to his forgetting to wear his belt. Even untidiness is complicated. With most of the behaviors on the continuum, the early behaviors fade as a child moves along in recovery. Recall, for example, that suicidal threats are actually more advanced on the continuum than the low affect, non-communicative behaviors that precede them. For some patients, the reading of social cues (a higher level skill) is not only flagrantly poor, but includes inattention to hygiene, perseverative mannerisms (picking at one's skin, for example), repeating the same phrases or anecdotes, or getting "stuck" on an idea (perseverative thinking). Therefore, some head injured students exhibit self-monitoring deficiencies across the whole spectrum, while others will show only the last group. One 16 year old girl observed that people often looked around while she talked and showed inattentiveness and lack of interest in what she was saying, a reasonable reaction to her conversation because she had so much trouble coming to the point and rambled slowly on and on. As she recovered, her attention to others' inattention was a significant mark of progress and she began to monitor her own dialogue more carefully.

Mood and Self-Esteem

In the very earliest stages of recovery, there is little self awareness. The metacognitive behavior of standing outside oneself and examining oneself is really a high level skill. We know that developmentally children demonstrate egocentric behavior until around the age of eight or nine, and then gradually develop more sensitivity toward others as they relinquish this self-centered view. Much of the recovery from coma resembles a passing through all the developmental periods from birth on. One emerges from unconsciousness to reclaim the skills once gained: walking, balance, talking, thinking, in just about the same order as when they were first learned.

In the newly recovering child, there is very little affect, or the child may move quickly to a very labile state in which crying and giggling may alternate. It will not be common to see a child in this condition in school, however, because these behaviors are observed very early after coma. The low affect may continue in a less severe form and be observed in those who return to school. As recovery progresses, awareness develops and is a sign of progress. When patients in the unit have begun to feel self-conscious and have resisted going out, the staff has viewed that as positive change, even while acknowledging that patients now face a new problem: depression and dissaffection with themselves. Overt fatigue and sadness mark this period, which often persists into the first year. Students respond to this with irritability and impatience with themselves and others. Teachers are likely to observe this period of low self-esteem and irritability in the returning students. To offset a student's fatigue, school personnel can provide rest periods, arrange the most demanding classes in the morning, or allow the student to attend a partial day.

A further stage of despair may develop for some students even while they are patients. Sometimes patients issue suicidal threats, and indeed want to commit suicide when they face the loss of mobility, independence, personal attractiveness and competence. Such despair affects the A student who now has trouble with work that had been easy; the swimming champ who wanted to go to college on a swimming scholarship (and could have) until the injury; the star football player on whom the whole team was counting to glorify their season; or the student with a long record of failure in school who has even more trouble learning now. Most of the suicidal statements have come from adolescents, a population that has a high rate of suicide *without* head injury, but younger children also express sadness and utter disappointment with themselves. The irony of this is that the ability to judge oneself and compare life now with then and project possibilities into the future are all signs of progress and recovery. The severely damaged child lacks this awareness. Teachers must have sensitivity to the child who has recovered enough to be aware but still hasn't recovered enough. This child returns to school with great self-doubt and hesitancy.

Professionals know that any suicide threat has to be taken seriously. Even though it may be certain that these head injured students couldn't organize themselves well enough to carry it out, the family and professional staff need to be alerted to the possibility. This is an opportune time to encourage counseling if the student isn't already receiving it and to explore other supportive services. For example, a number of former patients from the Kennedy unit participate in a therapy group that was organized expressly for the purpose of helping them with school and social readjustment, self-esteem, limitations and achievement.

In contrast, teachers may observe some students who have trouble directing their energies toward a particular task and whose mood is quite euphoric. Occasionally students giggle a little more than is expected, revealing a still present inability to exert control.

Thinking

It is important to keep in mind that the *qualitative* descriptions of cognitive behaviors are being discussed here in this elaboration of what teachers can expect to observe in head injured students. By the time these students arrive at school, they will have passed through many shadings of deficit from responding to sound or touch only, to responding to simple verbal commands and on up the ladder to an increasing understanding of language. At worst, teachers will face students who are easily distracted, lose their train of thought or focus very easily, seem rather "blank" or "out-of-it," and are very concrete and literal. As these students improve, their span of attention will increase but other peripheral activities in the classroom will compete strongly for attention. In this middle level, students experience much difficulty in coming to a point, organizing thought, categorizing information, or abstracting concepts. When individuals at this point in recovery are presented with a task that requires sorting or categorization, the disability is quickly obvious. One interesting tool for observing this is a sorting task in which an individual is asked to arrange a variety of objects in groups that go together. Such items are paper clips, pencils, string, crayons, a screwdriver, tape, a ball, or any items on hand. Can the student sort these into related groups? Or do the items get sorted by some concrete similarity such as color? Think of the levels of abstraction that are possible with such a task. Piaget's observation that a child in the early stages of thinking does not conceptualize houses as buildings or birds as animals gives a clearer idea of how limited a student's thinking will be in regard to what is being taught. Sixteen year olds can't be assigned to third grade classes, but sometimes that is the level of abstraction that students hold.

A student's further development along the continuum will reveal greater understanding of much classroom material but a remaining deficit on a higher level of abstraction such as in proverbs. Inference, drawing conclusions, and the ability to consolidate and integrate information are all likely to be compromised. This underlying deficit will override abstract thought and new learning in different ways.

For those students who enter school with the most severe deficits, the amount and speed of information will have to be reduced, whether it is in conversational, written or visual form. This is just an extension of the care given while in the hospital, when all staff are urged to speak more slowly in short sentences (not more loudly) and to give patients time to respond. Self-contained classrooms are helpful in reducing the amount of stimulation and in producing instruction geared to a low level of understanding. Students (and teachers) need a great deal of reassurance at this time that these deficits often improve very quickly. As improvement occurs, students will need exercises in ordering, sequencing, and establishing priority. Students do not need drill in the conventional sense of that word. Once they can order a series, they can move on to the next level of abstraction. Continued caution in presenting students with a heavy language component in their studies must be observed until teachers have evidence that it is no longer necessary. The subtleties of language are the last to arrive in recovery and the least likely to arrive at all.

Auditory Perception

Because auditory perception is an integral part of overall cognitive functioning, students show changing abilities to comprehend spoken language, and therefore face varying difficulty in tracking oral instruction and directions given in the classroom. Although maintaining attention in a large group is certain to be a component of that difficulty, short term memory is another, and processing of the language itself will reflect damage in the area of the brain that receives stimuli and in the areas that interpret the stimuli into meaning. Some degree of deficit is present in most patients, if only temporarily. At its worst, the deficit will put the student's performance several years below age level. A secondary student may have auditory comprehension comparable to a third grader. Clearly a teacher's directions to such a student will need to be simplified and repeated. Instruction will require clarification by use of familiar examples, visual presentations and individual instruction. Re-phrasing of questions and expectations will be necessary. As students improve, asking them to repeat what they thought they heard provides feedback to both teacher and student about whether understanding occurred.

Sensory and Perceptual Accomodations

It has been stated earlier that visual field cuts, including hemi-anopsia, are a possible outcome in head injury. Although only .04 percent of the Kennedy Institute population experienced such, teachers need to know whether this condition exists and should look for this information in the medical report sent to the school. Students and families usually know this as well. These students need to be seated in a position in class that provides optimum access to the visual field. For example, a student with a left field cut should be seated in the left area of the classroom so that most of what is viewed is to the right. These students may also need adapted physical education and will need to avoid classes with machinery, such as shop.

Writing Speed and Legibility

Some students arrive at school after their injuries with no ability to write. A permanent weakness will require that they change to the nondominant hand for writing. They will have to expend much time and effort to write well enough and fast enough for this change to be useful. Think about how long it might take to learn to use a nondominant hand skillfully enough to take notes in a lecture. Imagine the student's dilemma when an assignment is put on the board a few minutes before the class ends. Add to that the tension of trying to copy it before an early dismissal to reach the next class on time. This is an easy way of putting a student in a bind, whether it is a student who has to change hands in writing or one who will recover writing skill yet who still experiences much weakness. A student's fine motor ability may be weakened permanently so that even a substitute such as typing is not a viable solution.

Writing, therefore, whether a student has a total deficit or a mild one, requires much the same adaptation since it matters little whether a person writes very slowly or not at all. The effect is the same: The student has to have a scribe, a note taker, or some other way to review classroom instruction. The use of a good note taker's notes might be permitted or a tape recorder might be used, although as mentioned earlier, clear recording is hard to achieve. If students can learn to type, they might be encouraged to use a word processor or typewriter. Students will be severely penalized by written assignments and tests. Oral tests, multiple choice tests, assignments that require circling the answer, or other adaptations are needed for these students. Written tests need to be untimed.

Mathematics

During the early phases of the continuum there is much confusion in trying to recall math processes and number facts. At first, memory itself interferes with the recall of both, and language understanding affects the skill with which word problems are solved. As students improve, application problems often indicate that a student knows how to apply what has been learned or how to manipulate the concepts in new situations, but the memory for steps in lengthy procedures such as division of numbers by three divisors is sometimes so poor that the process is excruciating. Simple number facts may elude students at this time.

Students with severe loss of memory for number facts are often helped when they are given a more concrete way to manipulate information. At the lowest level of recall, fingermath helps move students beyond the need to recall facts in order to move on to conceptual work. Students need review and repeated exposure to content without unnecessary drill. There is no need to demand that a student calculate problems when the memory simply doesn't support such a demand. Calculators make more sense and reduce frustration. If a calculator is unavailable, a matrix of tables on 3×5 cards could serve as a reference. For the student who has forgotten the steps of a process, sample problems could be available. Steps might be presented the way they are in a text when the procedure is first presented. Some students will benefit from even more structure such as having the steps in different colors.

Abstract reasoning will be the last to appear, particularly in word problems. Students taking algebra may need to drop back to a basic math class or receive tutoring as they review the algebraic principles underlying the work being requested of them. Students who have geometry classes interrupted by the injury may have great difficulty in memorizing new theorems. These subjects need not be removed from the student's schedule, but teachers should try to assess just where the skill breaks down so they can review it, and tutoring or other support should be given so that a student can be maintained in the class.

Reading Speed and Comprehension

Students often re-enter school with low levels of reading comprehension and/or poor speed. As speed improves, single word identification and word attack skills often return to grade level while reading comprehension remains at least two grades below. At the upper levels of reading skill, comprehension may be close to grade level but speed often is reduced enough to be penalizing. Resource assistance is mandatory to help students comprehend content when they have inadequate decoding skills. Content has to be adapted and work must be untimed. Use of audiotapes or the use of a reader is sometimes helpful. Reading speed is often reduced for a long time into recovery. One high school senior in the Kennedy Institute population was permitted to take the SAT examinations untimed on the basis that her demonstration of what she knew would be hampered by a continuing deficit in reading speed.

Several reading strategies for meaningful learning have been reviewed by Pressley and Levin (1983) and are worth consideration for this population.

The REAP method (read, encode, annotate, ponder) by Eanet and Manzo (1976) emphasizes the role of annotation in demonstrating reading comprehension and in potential review of the material read. Having students restate others' ideas into their own words (encoding) is in itself useful, but when it is followed by a written summary (annotation), the combination provides an external record of comprehension as well as feedback, both to the student and teacher, about whether the essential ideas in a passage have been understood.

Eanet and Manzo suggest that annotation can take a number of other forms besides summaries (e.g., intention of author, major theme of passage, criticism of author's point of view, and so on). They believe that using the REAP procedure requires students to process information at higher inferential levels by reorganizing and manipulating the text.

This method serves two important purposes for head injured students. First, a written restatement of reading material provides students and teachers with a measure of comprehension that also can be used diagnostically by the teacher. Second, the practice of restating ideas and writing them down is likely to be a more effective technique for students with inefficient memory storage.

Another focus on reading comprehension studied by Earle (1969) is that of the structured overview, in which key terms and concepts are presented by the teacher prior to an assigned reading in an organized framework that highlights the relationships among the concepts. Although this method may be more effective in a subject like biology rather than English, a general instructional practice of presenting an outline or overview for head injured students helps them organize information, provides structure for note taking, and directs them toward the most important points of a lesson.

Another method chosen for its capacity to focus and direct attention is the Directed Reading and Thinking Activity (DRTA). Head injured students are likely to need reading assignments that direct attention to salient information, force searches for particular content and encourage relating that content to prior knowledge. Akin to "motivational" reading, Stauffer (1975) suggests activities that draw upon prior knowledge when reading and thinking about the meaning of materials. For example, a class is given the title or first paragraph or picture descriptive of the passage and is asked to predict the meaning of the passage by these clues. This activity elicits information about the students' familiarity with the subject, identification of key terminology and level of general understanding. This technique seems particularly relevant to head injured students because of its unique characteristic of drawing on relevant prior knowledge, since head injured students may indeed have that, and it may be more accessible than recently learned information. There is also additional benefit to linking new information with old as a way to remembering it more efficiently. In effect, this technique utilizes advance organizers by exploring the possible content before reading the passage.

ORIENTATION

By the time most students return to school, the most severe orientation problems have resolved themselves. It may be helpful to review how much orientation changes in patients to appreciate some of the residual difficulties. Patients usually experience moderate to severe disorientation as they emerge from coma. This period of disorientation and impaired memory storage constitutes posttraumatic amnesia. Sometimes confusion and amnesia create total disorientation. Patients may have trouble understanding where they are and why they are in a hospital. Most people have had the experience of being unable to recall for a few moments where they are upon waking. Think about how it might feel if that cloud of confusion did not lift. It is also common for patients to have momentary trouble remembering what day it is or, more frequently, the date. Posttraumatic amnesia persists for varying time periods with each head injured individual. Rehabilitation treatment often includes a daily orientation group meeting. In addition to the daily review of name, place, date and events, patients are asked to tell why they are in the hospital. Their knowledge about these events is quite superficial. For example, even though several members of one group were sitting in wheelchairs, no one thought there was a problem when asked if anyone there had any problems with walking. The loss of awareness seems a bit like being suspended in time or place. Walking is something most patients have always been able to do. The realization of being unable to do so, even temporarily, had not been incorporated into their view of themselves.

When students return to school, some confusion remains about finding their way around the building, particularly if it is a new building. A buddy is needed temporarily. Lasting disorientation is rare, although head injured students may have persistent problems with short term memory and visual-spatial orientation. It would seem that losing one's way is easily remedied by asking for directions, but the fact that the most reasonable and rational solutions are not always available to head injured students cannot be discounted. One mother tells of practicing for weeks a plan for traveling to another city with her head injured daughter. She thought she had covered all possibilities, stressing as an option that if her daughter became lost, she could always call a cab. But she hadn't told her how to do *that*, and her daughter walked the streets for 2 hours before finding someone she deemed safe enough to ask for help.

Chapter 7

Summary and Issues

It seems worth noting that over the course of 3 years of discussion with school officials about school placement and the needs of head injured students, teachers rarely asked any questions about what to expect or how to handle forthcoming problems. This is likely to be accounted for by two reasons: Teachers may not know *enough* about such injuries to know what they do not know or what to anticipate; second, there is a general tendency among teachers and administrators to avoid revealing any uncertainty about managing the educational domain. Usually head injured students have been perceived as students who could be provided for as well as any other student and therefore imminent problems have not been raised. Problems that have developed after school reentry have been presented more in the form of complaints about failure to carry out tasks or failure to comply with school rules rather than as problems the staff might have in understanding the student.

The following questions are ones teachers might be compelled to ask after gaining some familiarity with head injury:

Q: Are head injured students affected by noise and confusion?
A: Yes; students admit that even parties are difficult. Corridors and cafeterias are especially hazardous because to navigate

among many moving people requires the ability to predict where others will move and the ability to move quickly to avoid bumping into others. These students may be unable to correct course quickly enough and, in addition, often have poor motor coordination.

There is also a period of time close to the injury when individuals experience "internal noise," an aggravation caused by easy distraction, blurring of thoughts, associative thinking, poor memory and perplexibility. The patient is confounded and bewildered by an abundance of stimuli and incoming information to a damaged and irritated brain.

Q: Can head injured students participate in sports and physical education?

A: During the first year after injury, it is advisable they avoid contact sports and any activity with a high risk for hitting the head. The student's physician should re-evaluate the activity after that.

Physical education instructors can adapt most activities for handicapped students, so physical education ought to be included in the schedule.

Q: Is it all right for these students to take driver education classes?

A: Allowing students to participate in driver education classes leads them to anticipate driving after they have passed the written and road tests, whereas the actual ability to do so will also depend on their motor coordination, vision and judgment. These latter qualifications may yet be deficient in the first few years after injury. People do drive with vision field cuts, but generally only after learning to accommodate their restricted vision. Because passing the tests will give students the means to put strong pressure on their parents to allow use of the car (often against their better judgment), it is recommended that classes be deferred temporarily, or until the student's physician gives approval.

Q: Should head injured students wear helmets?

A: Wearing helmets inside school stigmatizes children, and usually they are unnecessary during school hours. If the student's balance is still unstable, a head injured student can be taught how to fall so as to protect the head. Sometimes administrators worry about liability, but if physical therapists and physicians do not prescribe a helmet, then administrators can relax. Promoting helmet use for cyclists of all ages, especially by capitalizing on the current glamour of racing clothes that includes a helmet, would serve a better purpose.

Q: Does this student have seizures or fits? If so, what should I do?

A: Seizures are common in 5 to 32 percent of head injured children depending on the severity of the injury. Teachers should be informed by the family or hospital personnel whether a student has seizures, how severe they are and what procedure to follow when they occur. This information can be retrieved by the school nurse who can advise the staff how to respond.

Q: Is it appropriate to point out untidiness and careless hygiene to a student?

A: Yes, just as would be done with any student. The reasons for uncleanliness ought to be ascertained first. Is there no hot water in the home? No supervision (e.g., parent working)? Inattention to detail due to the injury? (One head injured student forgot repeatedly to put on his belt after a wrestling class during first period. Obesity from hyperphagia combined with poor memory contributed to low hanging slacks which exposed the top of his buttocks, much to the staff's distress and his peers' amusement.) Supervision will need to be supplied at school and a student's self-care addressed privately. Someone (nurse, teacher, coach, gym teacher, guidance counselor) will need to supervise a shower and remind the student daily about what is needed. Sometimes a contract can be developed for showering at home. At any rate, supervising personnel must not be punitive, but remain matter-of-fact, stating what the problem is and how to change it.

Q: What supervision is needed during a fire drill?

A: If a student is in the classroom, no extra supervision is needed. If the student is out of the classroom (e.g., going to therapy or using the bathroom), someone should be responsible for finding that student and providing an escort out of the building.

Q: Can head injured students participate in industrial arts classes?

A: That will depend on fine motor deficits and safety judgment around mechanical or electrical equipment. The instructor for those classes or an occupational therapist may help assess the advisability of the student's attending those classes.

Q: Is it harmful to mention or refer to a student's accident? Will it revive bad memories, particularly if there was a death involved?

A: It is not uncommon for a student's relative or friend to die in the accident. Staff members at the Kennedy Institute were also most concerned when the first instance arose. T.J., a 16 year old, lost her mother and brother when an out-of-control vehicle hit the three of them as they walked along the sidewalk. Who would tell her and what would be the effect? The individual may be protected from early emotional pain. Initial cognitive and emotional impairment may severely limit emotional comprehension and experience. As part of the cognitive impairment, poor short term memory may prevent dwelling on the loss.

The emotional lability mentioned in Chapter 3 is a superficial response of silliness or crying that is generally unrelated to the topic being considered. It is not to be confused with the restoration of deep feelings.

Some general practices may be helpful in answering other questions not raised here:

- Try to keep the demands on head injured students consistent with what is expected of others, especially socially.
- When behavior is erratic or negative behaviors persist, look for a reason related to the injury (memory, poor orientation, and so forth); supply enough structure to correct the situation (a buddy, contracts, point system) rather than assume this student is unmotivated, recalcitrant, or stupid.
- Confront behavior in a nonjudgmental, matter-of-fact manner, pointing out what is appropriate or inappropriate and supplying alternative behavior.
- There is no need to be reticent about a head injury and open discussion with all students may promote more understanding among others and less embarrassment for the injured.

Sometimes individuals fear that head injury will be interpreted as craziness or retardation. Patients at the Kennedy
Institute are taught to acknowledge their injuries and to identify some of the problems they are experiencing.

- Ask for as much information as possible from the family,
  hospital, social worker, or anyone working professionally
  with this individual. Ask what to expect, what current problems people recognize, what is now different from before
  the injury, what is needed, how severe the injury is (e.g.,
  how many days of coma), the area of specific injury, what
  therapy needs still exist, and so on. Even though teachers
  are not responsible for all facets of recovery, having a lot of
  information helps fill in the global picture of this student.
- Stay in touch with therapists. Ask what carryover is needed
  in the classroom. Stay in touch with the family. Communication between school and home is more important than
  ever.

PROBLEMS FROM THE FAMILY'S POINT OF VIEW

By the time head injured students return to school, parents have
been through a lot. In those instances where children remain
very severely damaged, very deep grief is felt over the loss of
normal children, and perhaps parents also harbor some amount
of ambivalence about whether it would have been better after
all if their child had died. There is no closure for the grief
because there is still a living child. One parent, discussing his
predicament as a widowed father trying to manage a very difficult teenaged daughter, said eloquently, ''I used to pray to God
to spare my daughter's life. God answered my prayers but I didn't
know what I was going to get. Now, I've got to make the best
of things.'' Families need a lot of support from many sources,
but especially they need the cooperation and understanding of
their child's teachers.

In an informal questionnaire which explored the problems
that families encountered in resuming their child's school participation, parents experienced the following difficulties to some
extent:

- lack of teacher understanding

- uncooperative and insensitive mainstream teachers
- loss of friends for child, particularly during the transition to a new school or new classes; social isolation; rare invitations by friends
- parental isolation (e.g., one mother was no longer asked to volunteer at school; another felt avoided by parents of her child's friends)
- parental strain from working with children on homework
- class placement sometimes thought to be inappropriate

All emphasized their gratitude for support from teachers and its importance.

PROBLEMS FROM THE PROFESSIONAL'S POINT OF VIEW

The Maryland Head Injury Foundation has found that families experience much frustration in finding needed services in the community and in coordinating those services from a number of sources.

Shorter hospital admission followed by long periods of outpatient rehabilitation are a current trend. One of the main reasons for the shorter stay is the intense economic pressure to curtail hospital costs. Patients are now discharged when physicians think they are medically stable and when a multidisciplinary team determines that the family can adequately manage an outpatient program. This kind of rationale places a heavy burden on outpatient facilities that are sometimes ill-equipped to handle this type of patient.

Therapeutic services as a provision of Public Law 94-142 are an important resource for rehabilitation patients. Physical, occupational, speech and counseling therapies are provided to handicapped students as part of a comprehensive curriculum. Many communities otherwise lack these important services that only the school system can provide. In addition, special education provides the opportunity for a student to be followed in a multidisciplinary fashion, with participating services of education, occupational therapy (OT), physical therapy (PT), and speech and counseling cooperating in day-to-day management.

In this way, treatment continues in a centralized fashion and the opportunity exists for frequent reassessment as the patient's clinical and academic pictures change. A member of this educational team may be assigned the role of liaison with the hospital rehabilitation unit when it is necessary to work on specific problems in common. This person or a school social worker may fill the role of case manager to coordinate ongoing services throughout the community for the child and family.

Because of the need for multidisciplinary cooperation, it is beneficial to have needed services centralized in a single community agency. If the school system does not assume this function, then a community agency with as many services as possible is recommended. This concentration of services prevents unnecessary and difficult transportation, duplication of services, and inconsistent management due to unresolved differences in therapeutic approach. If division of services is unavoidable, the case manager's coordination is especially important in the long term treatment of a student with chronic head injury. There is frequently the need for many services and some of these services may be necessary for months or years. In addition, a sudden change in the patient's clinical picture in a particular area of deficit may influence management in other areas. Most important is that posttraumatic treatment of these deficits is not standard in any discipline. Therapists of various disciplines may operate according to theoretical formulations that are in pronounced disagreement to the strategies of other workers. If disagreements among therapists negatively affect a student's progress, then those involved from the various disciplines will want to convene to reassess the patient's clinical status and to come to a consensus about further therapeutic strategies. Teachers can make an important contribution here by submitting observations and records of classroom behavior and achievement.

Availability of these school-delivered services, including classroom instruction, is very uneven. Although the law is clear about what is due, systems vary in their ability to provide it. Funded positions sometimes remain unfilled for lack of available therapists.

Availability of classroom instruction depends on the coincidence of the injury with the school year. The critical period of recovery for a child injured in the spring generally falls in the summer—a bleak time to find services and schooling. The badly needed structure, routine, instruction and opportunities for socialization have to be put on hold until September, while immediate needs for therapies are attempted to be met here and there in the medical and private sectors. Appropriate day camp programs are almost nonexistent. One 15 year old was accepted in a public day camp program that was intended for much younger children with learning disabilities. He was given the role of "junior counselor." This very rewarding experience provided by sympathetic and willing camp directors was unique. Over 3 years of this study, little of that nature was available for Kennedy Institute patients. Most of the day camp or summer school programs offered by a few counties were for retarded children or were for remediation in subjects the student had recently failed. Although the remediation classes appear to meet the need, they are often too intensive and too brief for head injured students.

The classification of psychiatric disorders is currently under revision in an attempt to define diagnoses by criteria which stem from historical material and current phenomenologic research. Most of the posttraumatic psychiatric literature was written prior to attempts at standardization of diagnosis. The DSM III has attempted to group together organic diagnoses (psychologic or behavioral abnormalities associated with transient or permanent brain dysfunction). Terminology has been simplified with the proposal of operational definitions and criteria have been defined. The diagnosis "organic brain syndrome" is used to refer to a constellation of psychologic or behavioral signs and symptoms without reference to etiology. Ten organic brain syndromes are listed which include delirium, dementia, amnestic syndrome, organic hallucinosis, organic delusional syndrome, organic affective syndrome and organic personality syndrome. When the etiology of a particular organic brain syndrome has been clarified, then the syndrome is moved from the general designation "organic brain syndrome" to a more specific designation of organic mental disorder. This occurs when the clinical presentation, mode of onset, progression, duration, and nature of the underlying process are defined. For example, a number of organic abnormalities due to alcohol have been characterized. Alcohol withdrawal delirium, alcohol hallucinosis, alcohol amnestic disorder and dementia associated with alcoholism are specific organic mental disorders attributed to the toxic effects of alcohol on the central nervous system.

It is reasonable to assume that organic mental disorders attributed to pathologic effects of closed head injury will eventually be characterized. Thus closed head injury delirium, closed head injury hallucinosis, closed head injury amnestic disorder, and dementia associated with closed head injury will hopefully be elaborated in future editions of the DSM. Until then, it is necessary to fit patients into the more general organic diagnoses. These diagnoses, however, often do not fit well nor do they give an adequate clinical description of the problem. The posttraumatic psychiatric literature is still in a descriptive phase. Writers list and may describe psychiatric deficits, but there have been few attempts to follow these deficits prospectively. There are even fewer studies of intervention strategies. Some authors have attempted to group signs and symptoms into a specific illness or syndrome. A notable example has been to adapt the frontal lobe syndrome described after open injury to a group of symptoms that may follow closed head injury. Because the clinical psychiatric picture following closed head injury is often imprecise, different authors ascribe different symptoms to this closed head injury frontal lobe syndrome.

A lack of common terminology by the several disciplines involved in the study and treatment of mental disorders also confounds diagnosis and interdisciplinary communication. Psychiatrists, clinical psychologists, behavioral psychologists, social workers and educators have each developed a respective terminology, system of diagnosis and treatment modalities for their clients. Each group may use a different term to describe a certain ailment or the same term to describe different ailments. For example, early in the inception of the pediatric rehab team, the term "alert" was used by nurses to describe a state quite different from that used by the clinical psychologist. Many speech and language pathologists and occupational therapists utilize the Rancho Los Amigos Scale described earlier. However, this scale does not use medical terms such as "coma" or "posttraumatic amnesia," nor does it describe early common psychiatric features such as hallucinations or sleep/wake disturbances. A standard terminology would be useful in locating a patient on a continuum of recovery. Further, use of the term "coma" for evaluation of prognosis requires agreement among its users about how it is measured.

Differences in interpretation of behavior in adults and children contribute another obstacle to classifying psychiatric sequelae. The literature describes posttraumatic psychiatric dysfunction of the child as misbehavior and emotional disorder. Psychiatric dysfunction in the adult is viewed as personality change as well as emotional disorder. It is unclear whether behaviors of hyperactivity, aggressivity, and perseveration are equivalent to personality traits of impulsivity, explosiveness, and obstinacy, or whether posttraumatic disorders are different at different stages of development. It is also possible that a behavior or personality trait may pass unnoticed because it is not objectionable at a certain age. For example, the appearance of apathy in a formerly robust, overactive youngster is sometimes viewed as an improvement in behavior by parents. On the other hand, apathy or lack of motivation is a trait that may be poorly tolerated in a person of previous high function. A prospective study of injured children followed into adult life is needed to provide information concerning the continuity and the duration of these observed traits.

To summarize, two immediate needs in this area of posttraumatic psychiatric sequelae are for a standardized or common terminology and a simple classification of disorders. The community mental health movement has provided some impetus to multidisciplinary agreement to utilize the DSM III terminology and classification.

Appendix A

Glasgow Coma Scale

EYE OPENING
    Spontaneous   E4
    To Speech   3
    To Pain   2
    Nil   1
BEST MOTOR RESPONSE
    Obeys   M6
    Localizes   5
    Withdraws   4
    Abnormal flexion   3
    Extensor response   2
    Nil   1
VERBAL RESPONSE
    Oriented   V5
    Confused conversation   4
    Inappropriate words   3
    Incomprehensible sounds   2
    Nil   1

COMA SCORE $(E + M + V)$ = 3 to 15

Note. From *Management of head injuries* by B. Jennett and G. Teasdale, 1981, Philadelphia: F.A. Davis. Copyright 1981 by Jennett and Teasdale. Reprinted by permission.

Appendix B

Children's Orientation and Amnesia Test (COAT)

Name _____   Date of Test _____
Age _____ Sex   M   F   Day of the Week S M T W T F S
Date of Birth _____   Time   AM   PM
Diagnosis _____   Date of Injury _____

INSTRUCTIONS FOR EXAMINER: Begin by introducing yourself by name (e.g., "Dr. _____") and ask the child to be sure to remember your name. Points for correct responses (shown in parentheses after each question) are scored and entered in the columns on the extreme right side of the test form. Enter the total points accrued for the items in the lower right corner of the test form. Children ages 3 to 7 are administered only the General Orientation and Memory sections of the test. The entire test is administered to children ages 8 to 15.

General Orientation   Points:

1. What is your name? first (2) _____
   last (3) _____   (5) _____
2. How old are you? (3) _____ When is your birthday?
   month (1) _____ day (1) _____   (5) _____
3. Where do you live? city (3) _____
   state (2) _____   (5) _____
4. What is your father's name? (5) _____
   What is your mother's name? (5) _____ (10) _____
5. What school do you go to? (3) _____
   What grade are you in? (2) _____   (5) _____

6. Where are you now? (5) _____   (5) _____
   (May rephrase question: Are you at home now? Are
   you in the hospital? If rephrased, child must correctly answer both questions to receive credit.)
7. Is it daytime or nighttime? (5) _____   (5) _____
                              General Orientation Total   _____

Temporal Orientation

8. What time is it now? (5) _____   (5) _____
   (correct = 5; ½ hr. off = 4; 1 hr. off = 3; greater than
   1 hr. off = 2; 2 hrs. off = 1)
9. What day of the week is it? (5) _____   (5) _____
   (correct = 5; 1 off = 4; 2 off = 3; 3 off = 2; 4 off = 1)
10. What day of the month is it? (5) _____   (5) _____
    (correct = 5; 1 off = 4; 2 off = 3; 3 off = 2; 4 off = 1)
11. What is the month? (10) _____   (10) _____
    (correct = 10; 1 off = 7; 2 off = 4; 3 off = 1)
12. What is the year? (15) _____   (15) _____
    (correct = 15; 1 off = 10; 2 off = 5; 3 off = 1)
                              Temporal Orientation Total   _____

Memory

13. Say these numbers after me in the same order. (Discontinue when the child
    fails both series of digits at any length. Score 2 points if both digit series
    are correctly repeated; score 1 point if only 1 is correct.)

3	5 _____	35296	81493 _____	
58	42 _____	539418	724856 _____	
643	926 _____	8129365	4739128 _____	(14) _____
7216	3279 _____			

14. How many fingers am I holding up? 2 fingers
    (2) _____ 3 fingers (3) _____ 10 fingers (5) _____   (10) _____
15. Who is on Sesame Street? (10) _____   (10) _____
    (can substitute other major television show)
16. What is my name? (10) _____   (10) _____
                              Memory Total   _____
                              OVERALL TOTAL   _____

NOTE: (Question 5, General Orientation)

   If a child age 3 to 6 correctly states that he or she does not attend
   school, give full credit. For children enrolled in preschool, credit is
   given for stating the teacher's name in lieu of stating the grade.

Note. From "Assessment of posttraumatic amnesia in head injured children"
by L. Ewing-Cobbs, H.S. Levin, J.M. Fletcher, E.J. McLaughlin, D.G. McNeely,
J. Ewert, and D. Francis, February, 1984, paper presented to the International
Neuropsychological Society. Copyright 1984. Reprinted by permission.

Glossary

anomia: a naming impairment that is the most common linguistic deficit following closed head trauma. A test for naming ability as a component of oral expression is included in aphasia batteries.

aphasia: a term that includes various deficits in the expressive and receptive aspects of language. Aphasia may be diagnosed clinically or by means of a standardized battery of tests. The diagnosis in a child who has not yet attained mature language function may be difficult. Language impairment is common after severe closed head injury in children and adolescents. Some workers define this impairment as aphasia, while other workers view the bulk of this impairment as part of a global cognitive deficit that follows the injury.

ataxia: a failure of muscular coordination that results in impaired balance, tremors, and dysarthric speech. It is a common motor impairment following severe closed head injury, caused by damage to the cerebellum or to sensory tracts that regulate coordination of movement.

coma: a state of unconsciousness with limited behavioral responsiveness. The depth and duration of coma are important indicators of prognosis in closed head injury. Termination of coma is commonly measured by attainment of a simple command level by the patient.

computerized tomography or **CT scanning**: a rapid, non-invasive, X-ray method of visualizing the inside of an organ and the extent of its disease. The technique has been adapted for use with many organs, including the brain.

disinhibition: a lack of control that contributes to a number of maladaptive behaviors seen after head injury. These behaviors are often attributed to frontal lobe dysfunction and include carelessness in hygiene and dress, inappropriate words or acts, overtalkativeness, and hyperphagia. Disinhibition tends to lessen over time and may respond to conditioning methods.

dysarthria: a deficit in the oral-motor aspects of speech that include intonation. Dysarthria is often combined with an expressive or receptive language deficit.

edema: the excessive accumulation of fluid that occurs in the brain as a result of closed head injury. The acute mechanical and drug treatment of closed head injury aims to decrease formation of and to remove edema fluid.

electroencephalogram (EEG): a measure of brain electrical activity using a standard arrangement of electrodes attached to the scalp. The process is painless and is performed while the patient is in both the sleep and wake states. Abnormality is defined as deviation from normal patterns. EEG readings are often grossly abnormal for varying periods after head trauma. EEGs have not proved to be very helpful in the prediction of posttraumatic epilepsy.

Glasgow Coma Scale: a widely used, easily administered intensive care clinical scale that measures the depth and duration of unconsciousness. Three components (eye opening, verbal ability, and motor ability) are scored and then combined into a composite score from 3 to 15. A patient with an initial Glasgow Coma Scale of 8 or lower is usually admitted to a specialized intensive care unit.

hematoma: an abnormal blood collection which occurs when trauma damages cerebral blood vessels, diagnosed by CT scan. These blood collections cause damage by occupying space and causing pressure on adjacent structures. Most hematomas must be removed by neurosurgical procedures to prevent compromise of vital functions. Occasionally a small hematoma may be simply observed by sequential CT scan until resolution occurs or it is certain that its presence poses no danger.

hemiparesis: See **paresis**.

hemiplegia: See **paralysis**.

hydrocephalus: an abnormal amount of fluid in the ventricular system which may occur as a complication of closed head injury. The ventricles will appear dilated on CT scan. This condition must be distinguished from cerebral atrophy with secondary dilation of the ventricles. If hydrocephalus is diagnosed and is due to an obstruction, then the cerebrospinal fluid can be shunted from the ventricular system to a blood vessel to relieve the build up of fluid.

hypertension: elevation of systemic blood pressure. Hypertension is more common and tends to last longer in patients with histories of prolonged coma.

intracranial pressure (ICP): the exertion of force upon structures within the brain by a combination of intracellular and extracellular fluids. Maintenance of intracranial pressure in the normal range is a central focus of intensive care after closed head injury. Heightened ICP damages the brain by causing mechanical distortion, or displacement of cerebral structures or reduction in cerebral blood flow. ICP may be continuously monitored by devices that are inserted into the space surrounding the brain. Medication and other treatments may then be administered in response to pressure changes.

neurointensive care: multidisciplinary care of severe neurologic illnesses carried out in highly specialized clinical units in major medical centers. These units are characterized by a high staff-patient ratio, advanced technologic instruments, and wide experience in pharmacologic management.

neuropsychology: that branch of psychology that attempts to test different specific components of cognition by examining cognitive elements such as memory or visuoperceptual function or reaction time. Primarily, the neuropsychologist is interested in determining the site and mechanism of damage to specific functions.

paralysis: neurologic muscular weakness or dysfunction to the extent of immobility. With lack of movement, muscles begin to contract and become smaller or atrophic. Paralysis of the extremities on one side of the body is called hemiplegia. Paralysis of all four extremities is called quadriplegia.

paresis: muscle weakness secondary to damage to brain pathways regulating movement. Hemiparesis is weakness of the extremities on one side of the body. Quadriparesis is weakness of all four extremities. The cranial nerves in the head governing muscle movements of sensory organs may also become paretic (e.g., paresis of an eye muscle may result in strabismus).

persistent vegetative state: the most severe sequela of severe closed head injury, occurring in about 5 percent of survivors. Heart and lungs function independently in this condition. The patient may move limbs, swallow, and make sounds, or may have periods of apparent sleep and wakefulness while the EEG may show normal alpha rhythms. The patient remains in a state of behavioral unresponsiveness, however, with no indication of mental functioning.

posttraumatic amnesia: the period of time after head injury for which the patient has no continuous memories. This period consists of the coma and the period of anterograde amnesia, measured by sequential tests of orientation and memory.

posttraumatic epilepsy: a type of seizure disorder occurring in greater than 5 percent of patients who suffer head trauma. The more severe the injury, the greater the likelihood that seizures will appear. Seizures may consist of motor or sensory activity or emotional states or may be a combination of these.

severe closed head injury: blunt head injury occurs with blows that cause damage by impact but do not penetrate the brain or its protective covering. Closed head injury is more likely to result in unconsciousness than open head injury, while open head injury is more likely to result in introduction of infection. Severe closed head injury may be defined as injury resulting in 6 or more hours of unconsciousness.

ventricles: cavities inside the brain which form a system of passage for the cerebrospinal fluid that circulates over and inside the brain. The spinal fluid serves as a protective cushion and as a carrier of nutrients and wastes to and from the blood. Enlargement of the ventricles after head injury may indicate an obstruction to the flow of spinal fluid, or more commonly, an indication of diffuse loss of cerebral substance.

visuoperceptual function: a person's visual interpretation of shapes, sizes, distances, and locations of objects, as well as recognition of faces. The Bender Gestal Test and tests of facial recognition are instruments that evaluate visuoperceptual ability.

References

American Psychiatric Association. (1980). *Diagnostic and statistical manual of mental disorders* (3rd ed.). Washington, D.C.

Ausubel, D. (1960). The use of advanced organizers in the learning and retention of meaningful verbal material. *Journal of Educational Psychology, 51,* 267–272.

Black, P., Jeffries, J.J., Blumer, D., Wellner, A., and Walker, A.E. (1969). The posttraumatic syndrome in children. In A.E. Walker, W.F. Caveness, and M. Critchley (Eds.), *Late effects of head injury* (pp. 142–149). Springfield, IL: Charles C Thomas.

Bower, G.H. (1970). Analysis of a mnemonic device. *American Scientist, 58* (5), 496–510.

Brink, J.D., Garrett, A.L., Hale, W.R., Woo–Sam, J., and Nickel, V.L. (1970). Recovery of motor and intellectual function in children sustaining severe head injuries. *Developmental Medicine and Child Neurology, 12,* 565–571.

Brink, J.D., Imbus, C., and Woo-Sam, J. (1980). Physical recovery after severe closed head trauma in children and adolescents. *Journal of Pediatrics, 97,* 721–727.

Brown, A.L. (1975). The development of memory: knowing, knowing about knowing, and knowing how to know. In H.W. Reese and L.P. Lipsitt (Eds.), *Advances in Child Development and Behavior: Vol. 10* (pp. 104–146). New York: Academic Press.

Brown, G., Chadwick, O., Shaffer, D., Rutter, M., and Traub, M. (1981). A prospective study of children with head injuries: 3. Psychiatric sequelae. *Psychological Medicine, 11,* 63–78.

Bruce, D.A. (1983). Management of cerebral edema. *Pediatrics in Review, 4,* 217–224.

Bruce, D.A., Raphaely, R.C., Goldberg, A.I., Zimmerman, R.A., Bilaniuk, L.T., Schut, L., and Kuhl, D.E. (1979). Pathophysiology, treatment and outcome following severe head injury in children. *Child's Brain, 5,* 174–191.

Chadwick, O., Rutter, M., Brown, G., Shaffer, D., and Traub, M. (1981). A prospective study of children with head injuries: 2. Cognitive sequelae. *Psychological Medicine, 11,* 49–61.

Clark, R.G. (1975). *Manter and Gatz's essentials of clinical neuroanatomy and neurophysiology.* Philadelphia: F.A. Davis.

Crosby, E.C., Humphrey, T., and Lauer, E.W. (1962). *Correlative anatomy of the nervous system.* New York: The Macmillan Co.

Dillon, H., and Leopold, R.L. (1961). Children and the post-concussion syndrome. *Journal of the American Medical Association, 175,* 86–92.

Eanet, M.G. and Manzo, A.V. (1976). REAP: a strategy for improving reading/writing/study skills. *Journal of Reading, 19,* 647–652.

Earle, R.A. (1969). Reading and mathematics in the classroom. *International Reading Association Conference Papers, 14,* 162–172.

Eiben, C.F., Anderson, T.P., Lockman, L., Mathews, D.J., Dryja, R., Martin, J., Burrill, C., Gottesman, N., O'Brian, P., and Witte, L. (1984). Functional outcome of closed head injury in children and young adults. *Archives of Physical Medicine and Rehabilitation, 65,* 168–170.

Ewing-Cobbs, L., Levin, H.S., Fletcher, J.M., McLaughlin, E.J., McNeely, D.G., Ewert, J., and Francis, D. (1984, February). *Assessment of posttraumatic amnesia in head injured children.* Presented at International Neuropsychological Society, Houston, Texas.

Fahy, T.J., Irving, M.H., and Millac, P. (1967). Severe head injuries: a six year follow-up. *Lancet, ii,* 475–479.

Fell, J. (1982). *Program manager: fatal accident reporting system.* National Highway Traffic Safety Administration.

Flavell, J. (1970). Developmental studies of mediated memory. In H.W. Reese and L.P. Lipsitt (Eds.), *Advances in Child Development and Behavior: Vol. 5* (pp. 182–209). New York: Academic Press.

Gagne, R.M., and Briggs, L.J. (1979). *Principles of instructional design* (2nd ed.). New York: Holt, Rinehart, and Winston.

Gaidolfi, E., and Vignolo, L.A. (1980). Closed head injuries of school-age children: neuropsychological sequelae in early adulthood. *Italian Journal of Neurological Sciences, 1,* 65–73.

Gilchrist, E., and Wilkinson, M. (1979). Some factors determining prognosis in young people with severe head injuries. *Archives of Neurology, 36,* 355–359.

Granholm, L. and Srendgaard, N. (1972). Hydrocephalus following traumatic head injuries. *Scandinavian Journal of Rehabilitation Medicine, 4,* 31–34.

Gronwall, D., and Sampson, H. (1974). *Psychological effects of concussion.* Auckland, New Zealand: Auckland University Press.

Guthkelch, A.N. (1979). Posttraumatic amnesia, post-concussional symptoms and accident. *Acta Neurochirurgica* (Suppl. 28), 120–123.

Hagen, C. (1981, January). *Diagnosis and treatment of language disorders secondary to closed head injury.* Paper presented at the conference on Models and Techniques of Cognitive Rehabilitation, Indianapolis, IN.

Hawkins, J.D., Lloyd, A.D., Fletcher, G.I.C., and Hanka, R. (1976). Ventricular size following head injury: a clinicoradiological study. *Clinical Radiology, 27,* 279–289.

Healy, G.B. (1982). Hearing loss and vertigo secondary to head injury. *New England Journal of Medicine, 306,* 1029–1031.

Higashi, K., Sakata, Y., Hatano, M., Abiko, S., Ihara, K., Katayama, S., Wakuta, Y., Okamura, T., Ueda, H., Zenke, M., and Aoki, H. (1977). Epidemiological studies on patients with a persistent vegetative state. *Journal of Neurology, Neurosurgery, and Psychiatry, 40,* 876–885.

Hounsfield, G.N. (1973). Computerized transverse axial scan (tomography): 1. Description of system. *British Journal of Radiology, 46,* 1016–1022.

Jennett, B. and Plum, F. (1972). Persistent vegetative state after brain damage, *Lancet, i,* 734–737.

Jennett, B., and Teasdale, G. (1981). *Management of head injuries.* Philadelphia: F.A. Davis.

Jennett, B., Teasdale, G., Braakman, R., Minderhoud, J., and Knill-Jones, R. (1976). Predicting outcome in individual patients after severe head injury. *Lancet, i,* 1031–1034.

Kalsbeek, W.D., McLaurin, R.L., Harris III, B.S.H., and Miller, J.D. (1980). The national head and spinal cord injury survey: major findings. *Journal of Neurosurgery, 53,* 519–531.

Kirby, J.R. (1984). *Cognitive strategies and educational performance.* Orlando, FL: Academic Press, Inc.

Klonoff, H., Low, M.D., and Clark, C. (1977). Head injuries in children: a prospective five year follow-up. *Journal of Neurology, Neurosurgery and Psychiatry, 40,* 1211–1219.

Kolb, B. and Whishaw, I.O. (1980). *Fundamentals of human neuropsychology.* San Francisco: W.H. Freeman and Co.

Leigh, A.D. (1943). Defects of smell after head injury. *Lancet, i,* 38–40.

Levin, H.S., Benton, A.L., and Grossman, R.G. (1982). *Neurobehavioral consequences of closed head injury.* New York and Oxford, England: Oxford University Press.

Levin, H.S., and Eisenberg, H.M. (1979). Neuropsychological outcome of closed head injury in children and adolescents. *Child's Brain, 5,* 281–292.

Levin, H.S., and Grossman, R.G. (1978). Behavioral sequelae of closed head injury. *Archives of Neurology, 35,* 720–727.

Levin, H.S., Meyers, C.A., Grossman, R.G., and Sarwar, M. (1981). Ventricular enlargement after closed head injury. *Archives of Neurology, 38,* 623–629.

Levin, H.S., O'Donnell, V.M., and Grossman, R.G. (1979). The Galveston Orientation and Amnesia Test: A practical scale to assess cognition after head injury. *Journal of Nervous and Mental Disease, 167,* 675–684.

Lewin, W.S. (1965). Observations on prolonged unconsciousness after head injury. In J.N. Cumings and M. Kremer (Eds.), *Biochemical aspects of neurological disorders* (2nd series) (pp. 182–213). Oxford: Blackwell Scientific Publications.

Lewin, W., Marshall, T.F., and Roberts, A.H. (1979). Long-term outcome after severe head injury. *British Medical Journal, 2,* 1533–1538.

Lewis, D.O. (1985, June 21). Child delinquents who later commit murder have identifiable traits, study suggests. *Psychiatric News,* pp. 32–34.

Lewis, D.O., Shanok, S.S., and Balla, D.A. (1979). Perinatal difficulties, head and face trauma, and child abuse in the medical histories of seriously delinquent children. *American Journal of Psychiatry, 136,* 419–423.

Lieberthal, E.M. and Liberthal, B. (1979). *Complete book of fingermath.* New York: McGraw-Hill, Inc.

Lishman, W.A. (1968). Brain damage in relation to psychiatric disability after head injury. *British Journal of Psychiatry, 114,* 373–410.

Miller, C. (1985, March). Hope for coma patients? *Medical World News for Psychiatrists*, pp. 21–23.

Miller, R.M., and Groher, M.E. (1984). General treatment of neurologic swallowing disorders. In M.E. Groher (Ed.), *Dysphagia: Diagnosis and management* (pp. 113–132). Boston: Butterworths.

Morrell, R.M. (1984). Neurologic Disorders of Swallowing. In M.E. Groher (Ed.), *Dysphagia: Diagnosis and management* (pp. 37–58). Boston: Butterworths.

Murray, G.B. (1985, April). Psychiatric disorders secondary to complex partial seizures. *Drug Therapy*, pp. 21–26.

Ommaya, A.K. (1966). Trauma to the nervous system. *Annals of the Royal College of Surgeons of England*, 39, 317.

Overall, J.E., and Gorham, D.R. (1962). The brief psychiatric rating scale. *Psychological Reports*, 10, 799–812.

Plum, F., and Posner, J.B. (1966, 1980). *Diagnosis of stupor and coma* (1st and 3rd ed.). Philadelphia: F.A. Davis.

Potter, J.M. (1970). Head injuries. In F.J. Gillingham (Ed.), *Neurosurgery: Clinical Surgery: Vol. 16* (pp. 48–89). London: Butterworth.

Pressley, M., and Levin, J.R. (Eds.) (1983). *Cognitive strategy research. Educational Applications*. New York: Springer-Verlag.

Richardson, F. (1963). Some effects of severe head injury: a follow-up study of children and adolescents after protracted coma. *Developmenal Medicine and Child Neurology*, 5, 471–482.

Robbins, D.M., Beck, J.C., Pries, R., Jacobs, D., and Smith, C. (1983). Learning disability and neuropsychological impairment in adjudicated, unincarcerated male delinquents. *Journal of the American Academy of Child Psychiatry*, 22, 40–46.

Rosman, N.P., and Oppenheimer, E.Y. (1982). Posttraumatic epilepsy. *Pediatrics in Review*, 3, 221–225.

Russell, W.R. (1932). Cerebral involvement in head injury. *Brain*, 55, 549–603.

Rutherford, W.H., Merrett, J.D., and McDonald, J.R. (1977). Sequelae of concussion caused by minor head injury. *Lancet*, i, 1–4.

Rutter, M. (1981). Psychological sequelae of brain damage in children. *American Journal of Psychiatry*, 138, 1533–1544.

Sarno, M.T. (1980). The nature of verbal impairment after closed head injury. *Journal of Nervous and Mental Disease*, 168, 685–692.

Sieber, J. (1968, August). Paper presented at the UNESCO International Conference on Learning and the Educational Process, Stockholm.

Stauffer, H. (1975). New materials on the market. *Reading Teacher*, 28, 478–487.

Strain, P., and Kerr, M. (1981). *Mainstreaming of Children in Schools*. New York: Academic Press.

Tanhehco, J., and Kaplan, P.E. (1982). Physical and surgical rehabilitation of patient after 6-year coma. *Archives of Physical Medicine and Rehabilitation*, 63, 36–38.

Teasdale, G., and Jennett, B. (1974). Assessment of coma and impaired consciousness. *Lancet*, ii, 81–84.

Wohns, R.N.W., and Wyler, A.R. (1979). Prophylactic phenytoin in severe head injuries. *Journal of Neurosurgery*, 51, 507.

Young, B., Rapp, R., Brooks, W.H., Madauss, W., and Norton, J.A. (1979). Posttraumatic epilepsy prophylaxis. *Epilepsia*, 20, 671–681.

Annotated Bibliography

American Psychiatric Association (1980). *Diagnostic and statistical manual of mental disorders* (3rd ed.). Washington, DC. This manual is the product of a continuing effort to improve and standardize psychiatric diagnosis in the United States. It is a great improvement over previous editions of the manual. Specific criteria must be satisfied in order to fulfill a diagnosis. This manual is currently being used in all accredited psychiatric facilities as well as by many mental health professionals. The special educator uses a different set of terms to describe emotional and behavioral disability. This manual may provide a valuable addition to the library of the special educator treating head injured students with behavioral and emotional problems.

Boll, T.J., and Barth, J.T. (1981). Neuropsychology of brain damage in children. In S.B. Filskov and T.J. Boll (Eds.), *Handbook of clinical neuropsychology* (pp. 418–452). New York: John Wiley and Sons. This chapter describes the rationale for the use of neuropsychologic tests in childhood. Tests are divided according to the function tested. Merits of the individual tests are discussed and specific indications for the performance of these tests are described.

Brink, J.D., Garrett, A.L., Hale, W.R., Woo-Sam, J., and Nickel, V.L. (1970). Recovery of motor and intellectual function in children sustaining severe head injuries. *Developmental Medicine and Child Neurology, 12,* 565–571. This is an important follow-up study from the Rancho Los Amigos Hospital of children and adolescents rehabilitated after very severe injuries. It documents resultant severe intellectual deficits after prolonged coma. Children over age 10 had better cognitive recovery than children below age 10.

Brink, J.D., Imbus, C., and Woo-Sam, J. (1980). Physical recovery after severe closed head trauma in children and adolescents. *Journal of Pediatrics,* 97, 721–727. This follow-up study describes the motor and neurologic consequences of very severe head injury in rehabilitated children and adolescents. The study population is divided by physical levels of dependence and independence. Functional outcome groups are discussed according to the deficit patterns they exhibit.

Brooks, D.N., and McKinlay, W.W. (1983). Personality and behavioural change after severe blunt head injury—a relative's view. *Journal of Neurology, Neurosurgery, and Psychiatry,* 46, 336–344. This is an excellent article describing personality change in 55 severely head injured adults. Half of the patients' relatives reported personality change at 3 months and nearly two thirds reported change by 6 and 12 months. Most of these changes were in the direction of increasingly negative or unpleasant features in personality. Even when patients were not viewed as having an overall personality change, relatives still described increased temper and irritability and decreased energy and enthusiasm.

Brown, G., Chadwick, O., Shaffer, D., Rutter, M., and Traub, M. (1981). A prospective study of children with head injuries: 3. Psychiatric sequelae. *Psychological Medicine,* 11, 63–78. This is the third part of the prospective study of Rutter's group. This comprehensive $2\frac{1}{4}$ year follow-up study is the most informative work yet published in the area of childhood head injury. Posttraumatic psychiatric disturbances are described in this article. A PTA longer than one week increases the risk for posttraumatic disturbance. The signs and symptoms are the same as in the non–head injured population. A collection of symptoms described as social disinhibition may be unique to patients who have had closed head injury.

Bruce, D.A., Raphaely, R.C., Goldberg, A.I., Zimmerman, R.A., Bilaniuk, L.T., Schut, L., and Kuhl, D.E. (1979). Pathophysiology, treatment, and outcome following severe head injury in children. *Child's Brain,* 5, 174–191. This technical article by a pediatric neurosurgeon describes the mechanism of closed head injury in children and how child injury differs from adult injury. The concept of primary and secondary injury is explained. Current medical intensive care is described in a clear fashion. Optimistic survival figures from centers around the world are compared and discussed.

Chadwick, O., Rutter, M., Brown, G., Shaffer, D., and Traub, M. (1981). A prospective study of children with head injuries: 2. Cognitive sequelae. *Psychological Medicine,* 11, 49–61. This is the second article of a series by Rutter's group. Posttraumatic cognitive deficits are described in children with mild and severe head injuries. Persistent intellectual impairment was not seen after mild injury. The cognitive deficit after severe injury was in a dose response relationship with the degree of brain injury as measured by the duration of the PTA.

Chadwick, O., Rutter, M., Shaffer, D., and Shrout, P.E. (1981). A prospective study of children with head injuries: 4. Specific cognitive deficits. *Journal of Clinical Neuropsychology,* 3, 101–120. This paper focuses on the cognitive and neuropsychologic testing of Rutter's study populations and controls. Neuropsychologic tests were chosen to identify specific deficits not seen on the WISC. In most cases, children without deficits on the Performance Scale of the WISC also did not show deficits on the neuropsychologic battery. In a few cases, however, tests of speed of visuomotor or visuospatial functioning picked up deficits attributable to the head injury that occurred in children with normal scores on the WISC.

Christoffel, K.K., and Tanz, R. (1983). Motor vehicle injury in childhood. *Pediatrics in Review, 4,* 247–254. This is an excellent review of types of injury by age group. In addition to describing injury mechanisms for each age group, it gives helpful information about prevention. The value of seat belt usage is clearly documented.

Dillon, H., and Leopold, R.L. (1961). Children and the post-concussion syndrome. *Journal of the American Medical Association, 175,* 86–92. Post-traumatic behavioral changes are described in children who have been unconscious for brief periods. The authors state that behavioral changes in children are equivalent to post-concussive symptoms seen in adults. Forty-seven of 50 children showed personality changes and psychologic phenomena including increased aggressiveness, regression, withdrawal, and antisocial behavior. Thirty-seven of 50 children reported headache.

Gerring, J.P. (1985). The diagnosis, treatment, and rehabilitation of severe closed head injury. In A.N. O'Quinn (Ed.), *Management of chronic disorders of childhood* (pp. 179–224). Boston: G.K. Hall. This chapter describes intensive care and inpatient rehabilitation of children and adolescents at a major medical center. Psychosocial aspects of rehabilitation are emphasized. Unmet needs are brought to the attention of the reader.

Institute of Rehabilitation Medicine. (1982). *Working approaches to remediation of cognitive deficits in brain damaged persons* (Monograph 64). New York: New York University Medical Center. This monograph describes a representative system of cognitive rehabilitation currently in use with the adult head injured population. Deficits are defined and are addressed by modules that focus on improvement in a specific area. Although a number of these programs exist and are carefully organized and structured, there are not yet follow-up studies that demonstrate an improved outcome with participation.

Jennett, B., and Teasdale, G. (1981). *Management of head injuries.* Philadelphia: F.A. Davis. This is the comprehensive text on the epidemiology and current acute treatment of closed head injury. Medical issues are treated clearly and in detail. There is a continual focus on issues that influence prognosis and functional outcome. The authors also give thoughtful treatment to topics of severe disability, persistent vegetative state, and the effects of chronic disability on family functioning.

Kirby, John R. (Ed.) (1984). *Cognitive strategies and educational performance.* Orlando, FL: Academic Press, Inc. An exploration of the impact of cognitive strategies upon academic performance, this collection is particularly appropriate for its discussion of findings of the effects of executive processes, metacognition, student motivation, and cognitive planning on learning.

Klonoff, H., Low, M.D., and Clark, C. (1977). Head injuries in children: a prospective five year follow-up. *Journal of Neurology, Neurosurgery, and Psychiatry, 40,* 1211–1219. Klonoff followed a group of children with severe closed head injury and normal controls prospectively for 5 years. He used a comprehensive battery to follow neuropsychologic function, neurologic status, EEG status, and school progress. He divided his population into 131 children younger than 9 years old at the time of injury and 100 children older than 9 years. Recovery could be documented throughout the 5 year follow-up in the areas examined.

Levin, H.S., Benton, A.L., and Grossman, R.G. (1982). *Neurobehavioral consequences of closed head injury.* New York and Oxford, England: Oxford University Press. This comprehensive text describes cognitive and neuropsychologic consequences of closed head injury. The authors do a complete review of past and current research including many studies by the author. There is one chapter that reviews the research involving children. This book is an excellent reference text for current technical information.

Mahoney, W.J., D'Souza, B.J., Haller, J.A., Rogers, M.C., Epstein, M.H., Freeman, J.M. (1983). Long-term outcome of children with severe head trauma and prolonged coma. *Pediatrics, 71*, 756–762. This optimistic medical article follows 34 children with an average coma length of 15.5 days for a period of 9 months to 4 years. Follow-up evaluations are not thorough. Twenty-nine percent of the survivors were normal at follow-up. An additional 53 percent had mild cognitive or behavioral problems, but 61 percent of these had evidence of similar problems prior to the injury.

National Task Force on Special Education for Student and Youths with Traumatic Brain Injury. (1985). *An Educator's Manual*. Framingham, MA: National Head Injury Foundation, Inc. A very practical compilation of information about head injury and its ensuing effects on educational and psychosocial life, this manual also discusses cognitive rehabilitation and the current interest in the use of computers for such. There is also resource information such as state affiliations of the Foundation and publishers' educational materials.

Plum, F., and Posner, J.B. (1966). *Diagnosis of stupor and coma*. Philadelphia: F.A. Davis. This seminal text in the neurology of coma led to the present theories and techniques for neurointensive care. The text describes the signs and symptoms of coma and suggests therapeutic ways to influence these signs and symptoms. The Glasgow Coma Scale is based on certain of these significant signs that are easy to detect and to follow.

Rimel, R.W., Giordani, B., Barth, J.T., Boll, T.J., and Jane, J.A. (1981). Disability caused by minor head injury. *Neurosurgery, 9*, 223–228. This is an important paper describing the neuropsychologic deficits and symptom complaints 3 months after a history of unconsciousness of 20 minutes or less in 424 adult patients. Of patients employed prior to their accident, 34 percent were unemployed 3 months after injury. There is yet no comparable child study that documents functional disability and impaired neuropsychologic functioning 3 months after injury.

Rosman, N.P., and Oppenheimer, E.Y. (1982). Posttraumatic epilepsy. *Pediatrics in Review, 3*, 221–225. This practical article defines early and late posttraumatic epilepsy and risk factors for their occurrence. Treatment alternatives are discussed in detail. The authors discuss the prophylactic use of anti-convulsants after injury to prevent the development of a seizure disorder.

Rutter, M. (1967). A children's behaviour questionnaire for completion by teachers: preliminary findings. *Journal of Child Psychology and Psychiatry, 8*, 1–11. A short behavior questionnaire describing behavior occurring in a school situation is described. This scale consisting of 26 items can be used to discriminate between different types of behavioral or emotional disorder. Good re-test inter-rater reliability was demonstrated. Such a scale has been useful in the documentation of posttraumatic psychiatric problems.

Rutter, M. (1981). Psychological sequelae of brain damage in children. *American Journal of Psychiatry, 138*, 1533–1544. Rutter reviews studies of psychologic deficits following head injury in children. He defines several risk factors for the development of psychologic problems. He also discusses the types of psychiatric disorder associated with brain damage. This is an excellent review article.

Rutter, M., Chadwick, O., Shaffer, D., and Brown, G. (1980). A prospective study of children with head injuries: 1. Design and methods. *Psychological Medicine, 10,* 633–645. Rutter and his group in London followed head injured children prospectively for more than 2 years. The study used orthopedic controls, a population of children with mild head injury, and a population of children with severe head injury. These children were followed with carefully selected test batteries at periods of 4 months, 1 year, and $2\frac{1}{4}$ years following injury. The authors' careful methodology is discussed in detail.

Sarno, M.T. (1980). The nature of verbal impairment after closed head injury. *Journal of Nervous and Mental Diseases, 168,* 685–692. An aphasia battery was administered to adults from 3 weeks to 8 years after severe head injury (median 27 weeks). No patient was spared some degree of verbal impairment. Thirty-two percent of 56 patients had aphasia, 38 percent had motor dysarthria and 30 percent had subclinical aphasia.

Shaffer, D., Bijur, P., Chadwick, O.F.D., and Rutter, M.L. (1980). Head injury and later reading disability. *Journal of the American Academy of Child Psychiatry, 19,* 592–610. Reading disability was evaluated in 118 children with a history of compound depressed skull fractures. Severe reading disability was significantly associated with a history of posttraumatic cerebral edema. Severe reading disability was also related to duration of coma in children injured before age 8 and to posttraumatic epilepsy in boys but not girls.

Author Index

Subject Index

NOTES

NOTES